Aromatherapy
FOR EVERYONE

SECOND EDITION

A PRACTICAL AND EASY-TO-USE GUIDE TO
UNLOCKING THE POWERS OF ESSENTIAL OILS

Mary Shipley

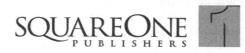

SQUAREONE
PUBLISHERS

The information and advice contained in this book are based upon the research and the personal and professional experiences of the author. They are not intended as a substitute for consulting with a healthcare professional. The publisher and author are not responsible for any adverse effects or consequences resulting from the use of any of the suggestions or procedures discussed in this book. All matters pertaining to your physical health should be supervised by a healthcare professional. It is a sign of wisdom, not cowardice, to seek a second or third opinion.

IN-HOUSE EDITOR: Michael Weatherhead
COVER DESIGNER: Jeannie Tudor
TYPESETTER: Gary A. Rosenberg

Square One Publishers
115 Herricks Road
Garden City Park, NY 11040
(516) 535-2010 • (877) 900-BOOK
www.squareonepublishers.com

Photographs reprinted by permission of Steven Foster.

Library of Congress Cataloging-in-Publication Data
Names: Shipley, Mary, author.
Title: Aromatherapy for everyone : a practical and easy-to-use guide to
  unlocking the powers of essential oils / Mary Shipley.
Description: Second [edition]. | Garden City Park, NY : Square One
  Publishers, [2019] | Revision of Aromatherapy for everyone / PJ Pierson
  and Mary Shipley ; [photographs by Steven Foster]. c2004. | Includes
  bibliographical references and index.
Identifiers: LCCN 2018010331 (print) | LCCN 2018011043 (ebook) | ISBN
  9780757054730 | ISBN 9780757004735 (pbk. : alk. paper)
Subjects: LCSH: Aromatherapy. | Essences and essential oils. | Vegetable oils.
Classification: LCC RM666.A68 (ebook) | LCC RM666.A68 P54 2019 (print) | DDC
  615.3/219—dc23

Printed in India

10   9   8   7   6   5   4   3   2   1

Contents

Introduction, 1

The Power of Aromatherapy, 3

Getting Started, 9

Becoming an Aroma Pro, 15

Your Guide to the Many Uses
of Essential Oils, 19

Allspice, 34

Anise Seed, 36

Balsam Fir Needle, 38

Basil, 40

Bergamot, 42

Black Pepper, 44

Camphor, 46

Carrot Seed, 48

Cassia, 50

Cedarwood, Atlas, 52

Cedarwood, Virginian, 54

Chamomile, Maroc, 56

Chamomile, Roman, 58

Cinnamon, 60

Citronella, 62

Clove, 64

Cypress, 66

Eucalyptus, Blue Gum, 68

Eucalyptus, Lemon, 70

Eucalyptus, Narrow-Leaved
Peppermint, 72

Frankincense, 74

Geranium, 82

Ginger, 84

Grapefruit, 86

Helichrysum, 88

Hyssop, 90

Jasmine, 92

Juniper Berry, 94   Pine Needle, 126

Lavender, 96   Rose, Cabbage, 128

Lavender, Spike, 98   Rose, Damask, 130

Lemon, 100   Rosemary, 132

Lemongrass, 102   Rosewood, 134

Lime, 104   Sage, 136

Marjoram, 106   Sage, Clary, 138

Myrrh, 108   Sandalwood, 140

Neroli, 110   Spearmint, 142

Nutmeg, 112   Tangerine, 144

Orange, 114   Tea Tree, 146

Oregano, 116   Thyme, 148

Palmarosa, 118   Vanilla, 150

Patchouli, 120   Vetiver, 152

Pennyroyal, 122   Wintergreen, 154

Peppermint, 124   Ylang-Ylang, 156

Resources, 159

References, 161

About the Author, 163

Index, 165

To Ann, J.T., Gwendolyn, and Sabrina,
for their love and support.

Introduction

The use of essential oils—or, as it is known today, aromatherapy —is appealing because of their user-friendly nature, versatility, and sensual properties. It has actually been around for centuries. People derive not only a great deal of pleasure from the use of these oils but also myriad health benefits.

Aromatherapy is a noninvasive way to take control of your health. Used in addition to other practices such as traditional Western medicine, yoga, meditation, diet, exercise, or holistic medicine, aromatherapy can strengthen your overall well-being and vitality. Because of aromatherapy's growing acceptance in the United States, essential oils are now available almost anywhere you look. This is both good and bad news. Good, as it is now easier for you to incorporate aromatherapy into your life. Bad, as essential oils, for the most part, don't come with instructions.

This book aims to demystify aromatherapy by explaining its history and usage. It covers the basic essential oils, including their aromatic characteristics and therapeutic properties. It also points out how to choose a quality essential oil and helps you pick out a starter kit. You'll also learn about combining oils for synergistic blends and the different ways aromatherapy may be incorporated into your life.

The power of aromatherapy can strengthen you both physically and mentally. Many people have already experienced this power for themselves, and now you can learn how to do so, too, by using this easy-to-understand guide. After reading this book, you'll find yourself excited about the positive changes you can make in your life through aromatherapy.

With a little bit of instruction, you'll be able to safely and confidently integrate essential oils into your everyday routine and discover a "scentsational" new lifestyle to embrace and enjoy.

The Power of Aromatherapy

Aromatherapy. You may not know exactly what it is, but you can't escape it. Everywhere you turn, there is a plethora of scented candles, oils, sprays, and incense all claiming to be good for your health and well-being. "Smell this and feel calm!" "Light this, and light his fire!" "Rub this scented lotion on your skin and reenergize your spirit!" Sounds like a bunch of nonsense just to sell products, doesn't it?

Strangely enough, it's not nonsense. In fact, there is more to aromatherapy than meets the nose. The use of scent to alter health and well-being for the better has been around for centuries. Now science has confirmed what men and women have practiced for generations: Scents have the ability to promote good physical, mental, and spiritual health. But how do you include aromatherapy in your everyday life? Is it easy? Does it make sense? And what exactly is it, anyway? This book will answer these questions and more. Armed with the answers, you can change your life—and your health—for the better!

THE BASIS OF AROMATHERAPY

Have you ever been in a funk and then smelled something wonderful, like lavender or citrus, and suddenly felt better? That's the basis of aromatherapy. Essentially aromatherapy is a gentle, noninvasive, natural healing art that utilizes the scents of essential oils to promote general well-being. While essential oils do, in fact, have medicinal properties, the simple act of smelling an essential oil can uplift the spirit, which can positively change feelings and outlook.

3

Aromatherapy's power lies in its ability to stimulate the imagination and generate an almost instant sense of joy or peace. And, unlike other therapies, such as acupuncture or traditional Western methods, aromatherapy is noninvasive. This means it does not involve needles or taking anything internally. It's also portable, so if you are dealing with problems such as stress, anxiety, headaches, or migraines, just take the applicable essential oil with you and you'll have help right at the tip of your nose at all times.

Don't let all that New Age talk fool you: Aromatherapy is not just a touchy-feely type of practice; there is most definitely science behind it. Aromatherapy falls under a fairly new science called psychoneuroimmunology, which studies the interaction among the psychological, neurological, and immunological systems. In layman's terms, psychoneuroimmunology looks at the effects of both positive and negative experiences on the immune system and the psyche. Science has confirmed that pleasurable experiences, such as breathing in a pleasant aroma or receiving a pampering massage, actually strengthen the body's immune system and uplift the spirit. Conversely, unpleasant things, like unhappiness or stale air, lower the body's resistance to disease and also dull the spirit. So, incorporating aromatherapy into your daily activities can actually help bolster your immune system and promote a positive, clear outlook on life.

You may have heard of holistic medicine, which looks at the causes and prevention of illness and not just symptoms of poor health. It's a whole-body approach to well-being—one that gives you responsibility and a certain amount of control over your health. Aromatherapy is part of holistic medicine. When married to a healthy diet and lifestyle, it's a fabulous, sensual, and creative way to keep on top of your health.

When Did Aromatherapy Arrive on the Scene?

The way aromatherapy is all the talk these days, you'd think it was a brand new concept in health and wellness. It's not. It's almost as old as civilization itself.

While there is reason to believe that the use of aromatics has been in place since the dawn of mankind, physical evidence dates back to the ancient Egyptians. Clay tablets have been found that mark the importation of cedarwood and cypress into Egypt and confirm the role essential oils played in international trade. Egyptian high priests also recorded the many uses of essential oils on papyrus. One intriguing fact is that Imhotep, King Zoser's chief architect, renowned physician and astronomer, is also known as "the grandfather of aromatherapy." This great physician is credited with significant advances in medical knowledge. He regularly incorporated the use of aromatics into his practice.

Other cultures have used aromatics as well. The Chinese used aromatic herbs and massage well before the birth of Christ. The Indian therapy known as Ayurvedic medicine utilizes massage techniques, pressure points, and essential oils to bring about good health. Hippocrates, the Greek physician known as the "Father of Medicine," also promoted daily use of aromatic baths and massage. These are just a few historical examples. The list also includes ancient Romans and various religious orders of the Middle Ages and continues through the centuries to these modern times.

How Do Aromatics Work?

It's not enough to know that aromatherapy has been around for ages, we also want to know how aromatics work. It doesn't seem possible that something as simple as the soothing smell of an essential oil could work wonders on health and well-being. Yet it is possible because it utilizes our strongest sense: smell.

Of all five senses, sense of smell hits the brain first. Faster than a speeding bullet, it's the "Superman of senses," with a direct path to the brain. Unlike many of our other senses, the olfactory system's nerve fibers do not pass through the "switching station" known as the dorsal thalamus. Instead, these nerve fibers run directly to the limbic area of the brain, which connects to the thalamus and neocortex. While these words may not have any meaning to you, this bit of information is important because it refers to the way in which aromas are able to affect conscious thought and reactions. The limbic system links directly to memories, learned responses, emotions, and feelings.

Even though the olfactory system is linked directly to the brain, it also involves other systems of the body. For example, someone breathing in an essential oil like peppermint absorbs it not only through the nasal cavity but also through much of the respiratory tract. This causes

5

the essential oil's molecules to pass into the body's circulatory system, increasing its benefits.

There is also an additional, sensual way to engage in aromatherapy: through the skin. This is done usually through massage, which has three very distinct beneficial aspects: touch, smell, and absorption. Essential oils can also be used in the bathtub, another relaxing and pampering activity. Besides the lovely scent essential oils produce when rubbed into the skin, their extremely small molecules pass through the epidermis to the dermis, the layer of the skin that gives skin its pliability. From there, the molecules pass into capillaries and journey through the rest of the circulatory system.

The body is not harmed by absorbing essential oils. The oils are expelled from the body in a variety of natural ways, like sweat, exhalation, and so on. The length of time it takes to expel these oils varies from three to fourteen hours, depending on the health of the body. Essential oils may come with warnings, of course, such as not to use them directly on the eyes or delicate mucous membranes of the body.

How Do I Use Essential Oils?

Aromatherapy is a user-friendly practice, so there is no excuse to shy away from it. Once you understand a few basics, the use of essential oils to attain a healthier, happier life is easy. While we have touched upon a few ways essential oils can be used, in the following chapters you'll discover how to get the most out of aromatherapy.

For solo artists (those of you who like to do things on your own), aromatherapy through scent is the way to go. For example, we know that peppermint is good for the digestive system, but did you know that smelling it will get you quicker relief than ingesting it? It's true! A 1963 Japanese experiment discovered this result. There are several ways to use scent, and one of the best and most common ways is through a diffuser. So, while opening a bottle of essential oil and taking a big whiff can be of some help, a diffuser emits the scent continuously, creating a pleasant, aromatic healing environment.

Some benefits, however, are best received through skin application. For instance, ginger oil, known for its bone-healing properties, can be applied directly to a small broken appendage, such as a toe. (Of course, this is in addition to Western therapy, which may include a splint of some sort.) Keep in mind that essential oils are highly concentrated oils. Make sure you carefully read the manufacturer's instructions for proper usage. Very few essential oils should be applied to the skin or ingested at full strength. Most require dilution, and some should not be used on the skin or ingested at all.

For those who like to share everything with family, friends, or loved ones, massage may be the therapy they are most drawn to. Touch itself is nurturing and healing. Massage can be doubly so when coupled with essential oils. When using an essential oil during massage, it's important to add it to what's known as carrier oil. This dilutes the essential oil somewhat and makes it last longer. The general rule is to add anywhere from 1 to 30 drops to 1 ounce of quality carrier oil.

Inhalation, direct application, and massage are among the most common ways to use essential oils, but there are many other ways as well. Some other uses of essential oils include but aren't limited to facial tonics, hot tubs, potpourri, humidifiers, mouthwash, perfume, sitz baths, face and body sprays, and creams and lotions. Once you start using aromatherapy, you'll find it fits into many different aspects of your lifestyle!

Getting Started

The great thing about essential oils is that they are remarkably safe and easy to use. Plus, they have a wide variety of every-day applications. They can be enjoyed for their pleasant aromas alone or used for their therapeutic value. Perhaps the whole spectrum of their soothing and healing properties is what appeals to you. No matter what aspect of aromatherapy you find attractive, there are a few simple yet essential things to know before you get started.

MEET THE AROMA FAMILIES

While you can most definitely start out with one essential oil and branch out from there, you may want to make yourself a starter kit. This basic kit would include at least one essential oil from each aroma "family," so that you can get more benefits from your personal aroma-therapy program. Plus, the advantages of essential oils often increase when blended with other oils.

There are eight families of aromas, and some essential oils may be classified under several families due to the complexity of their chemical structures.

- **Camphoraceous,** which includes camphor, eucalyptus, peppermint, rosemary, and tea tree.

- **Citrus,** which includes bergamot, citronella, grapefruit, lemon, lime, orange, and tangerine.

- **Earthy,** which includes patchouli.

- **Floral,** which includes chamomile, geranium, lavender, neroli, and ylang-ylang.

9

- **Herbaceous,** which includes basil, chamomile, clary sage, hyssop, lavender, and rosemary.

- **Resinous,** which includes frankincense and myrrh.

- **Spicy,** which includes allspice, anise seed, cinnamon, clove, ginger, and nutmeg.

- **Woody,** which includes cedarwood, juniper berry, pine needle, and sandalwood.

Starting with eight essential oils may sound overwhelming. It's acceptable to begin with fewer, but it's a good idea to start with at least two: lavender and eucalyptus. These are fabulous starter oils because they offer a broad range of health benefits and blend well together.

In choosing your oils, it's important to choose scents you enjoy. If a scent turns you off, you may not get the full benefit of that particular aroma. Additionally, because these oils are concentrated, they may smell stronger than you had first anticipated. This is where blending comes in handy. When compatible essential oils are mixed together, the scent can become more delicate and inviting.

The most important thing to remember is that there is no wrong choice in aromatherapy. Choose the oils that make your senses happy and you'll do just fine.

BASIC AROMATIC RECIPES AND APPLICATIONS

There are many ways to use essential oils. Following are some basic methods of use. The following recipes are general. For example, while the bath section suggests using 4 to 8 drops of essential oil, some essential oils are stronger than others, so maybe only 2 drops would be required. Therefore, once you've decided which oil you'd like to use, consult its individual entry for more specific guidelines.

Aromatic Bath

Essential oils can be added to bath water for pleasure alone or for therapeutic reasons. Either way, a long, luxurious soak in aromatic bath water is a treat for all your senses. The basic rule of thumb is to add

4 to 8 drops of essential oil to 1 tablespoon of a foaming product such as shower gel, shampoo, or Castile soap. The foaming product acts as an emulsifier, allowing the essential oil to be dispersed properly in the water and preventing it from floating on the surface. Once the bath is ready, add the mixture to the water and use your hand to agitate the water so that the oil is well dispersed. (As essential oils can make a tub slippery, add your mixture near the faucet area.)

Foot or Hand Bath

People with arthritis, rheumatism, athlete's foot, or other skin problems can benefit from hand or foot baths. Use a bowl or small tub big enough for your appendages. Make sure the water isn't too hot; it must be comfortable enough so that your hands or feet can enjoy generous soak time. Add 5 to 6 drops of the appropriate essential oil to 1 tablespoon of a foaming product such as shower gel, shampoo, or Castile soap, which acts as an emulsifier. Add the mixture to the bowl or tub and use your hand to agitate the water so that the oil is well dispersed. Next, place either your feet or hands in the bowl and soak them for about ten to fifteen minutes. After the soak, dry skin off completely. For added benefit, add a few drops of the same essential oil to carrier oil and massage into skin.

Aromatic Shower

Essential oils used with warm running water will vaporize the scent. A wonderful wake-up treatment using essential oils in a shower makes perfect sense. Choose an invigorating scent and after washing place 2 to 3 drops on a clean cloth or sponge and rub briskly all over your body. If using on your face, rub gently. Rinse as normal.

Sauna

The sauna is a wonderful appliance and offers a treat for both body and skin. The benefits of a sauna can be increased when an essential oil is added to the mix. Add just 2 drops of essential oil to approximately half a quart of water and throw it on the heat source. Do not use more than 2 drops, as more than this amount could be overpowering. (Caution: Avoid using sweet-smelling aromas, as they may cause nausea or headache when inhaled in such a tightly enclosed space. Rose, geranium, and ylang-ylang are three to avoid; eucalyptus, lemon, peppermint, and pine needle are four to use.

Hot or Cold Compress

There's nothing quite like a compress to help ease muscle aches, muscle sprains, or bruises. They also help reduce pain and congestion in internal organs. It's important to know when to use each, of course. A cold compress is best for recent injuries (sprains, bruises, swellings, or inflammation), headaches, migraines, or fever. A hot compress is best for old injuries, muscle aches, toothache, menstrual cramps, cystitis, boils, or abscesses. Additionally, some people with migraines may prefer a hot compress to a cold one.

To make a hot compress, add a few drops of the appropriate essential oil to a bowl of hot (not boiling) water. Take a clean cloth or bandage and soak it in the mixture. Wring out the excess and place over the affected area. Repeat as often as needed. A cold compress is made in a similar manner, except using your choice of cold or ice water.

Steam Inhalation

This is a wonderful way to clear the lungs and sinuses of congestion and infection. Add 2 to 3 drops of the applicable essential oil to a bowl of steaming hot water. Place your face over the bowl, drape a towel over your head, and breathe normally. Do this for a few minutes and then rest. You can repeat these steps a few times in a row, but discontinue this practice if you feel any discomfort. This particular method directly affects the respiratory tract and blood supply, so you may experience relief quickly after employing it.

Direct Application

Even though essential oils are natural and have a long history of safe use, they are highly concentrated botanical oils, so you should use them with common sense. While experienced aromatherapists and reflexologists often practice neat application—that is using the oil only—individuals just starting to explore the wonderful world of aromatherapy should exercise caution. Essential oils may be inhaled directly from the bottle, and some people like to add a few drops to a handkerchief for convenience.

Massage

The basic rule is to add 2 to 3 drops to 1 ounce of carrier oil and massage into affected areas. As some essential oils are stronger than others, it would be wise to consult the entry for your specific essential oil of choice before proceeding.

Gargle or Mouthwash

Some essential oils have the ability to fight bad breath, reduce the pain of a toothache, and soothe sore throats. The best way to attack these health challenges is through a gargle or mouthwash. A simple way to make one is to add 1 drop of applicable essential oil to 2 teaspoons of apple cider vinegar in a glass. Stir well to disperse the oil. Fill the glass with warm water and stir again. Gargle or rinse with the mixture. Use twice daily.

Diffusion

Two of the most popular and simple diffusers are the scent diffuser and the particle diffuser. A common scent diffuser is the lamp ring, or light bulb ring, which is made to sit on top of a light bulb. It uses the heat of the bulb to vaporize the oil's scent into the air. Usually 2 to 3 drops of oil is all that is needed for a scent diffuser. A particle diffuser is a little more advanced. It is usually an electronic appliance similar to a humidifier to which you would add a specified amount of oil. The oil would then be diffused into the air. Examples of particle diffusers include nebulizers and ultrasonic diffusers. Scent diffusers diffuse only the aroma of an oil into the air, while particle diffusers offer greater therapeutic benefit by actually diffusing oil particles into the air. (Caution: Never place oil directly on a hot light bulb. Never leave any diffuser operating unattended. Always follow manufacturer's instructions.)

BE CREATIVE

These are just a few fun and easy ways to use essential oils. You can also add essential oils to scent-free creams, lotions, shampoos, conditioners, or massage oils. Some people add them to the dishwasher or washing machine, and some even place a drop or two on a washcloth and add the washcloth to the dryer. Be creative and make up your own ways to employ these wonderful oils!

Becoming
an Aroma Pro

Now that you are familiar with the history and use of essential oils, it's time to get acquainted with the oils themselves. The following pages will introduce some of the most beloved and useful oils available today. After reading their descriptions, therapeutic uses, and benefits, you'll be able to decide which ones you want in your aromatherapy home kit. The helpful reference guide found in the next section (see page 19) will allow you to match your problem or need to the applicable essential oils that may be used in aromatherapy.

When choosing oils, think first about what you want the aromatics to do for you. For example, perhaps you lead a stressful lifestyle and crave serenity. A calming oil such as lavender would be a good option with which to begin. This one oil may not be enough, though, as anyone who leads a stressful lifestyle is probably in need of more energy as well. In this case, orange or any other citrus oil would be an optimal choice to add to your kit. Not only will it work to recharge your energy, but it will also blend well with lavender. As you read about the oils, be sure to check out the "Mixes Well with" section of each entry. Doing so will help you endow your home kit with synergy.

Secondly, be sure to get aromatics you enjoy, otherwise you may not experience their complete powers. For instance, rose oil is a strong aromatic. It is great for skin care and emotional balance. If you don't like the scent of roses, however, then your body won't respond as favorably as it might to an essential oil that has a scent you find pleasing. This is true because scent is very subjective, and one reason aromatherapy works is because it builds on what already appeals to and pleases you.

Finally, be sure to read the safety information provided. While the essential oils listed in this book are perfectly safe for home use, some come with special precautions, especially if you have been diagnosed with certain medical conditions. Additionally, as essential oils are highly concentrated, it's always a good idea to mix any essential oil with carrier oil before applying on skin. And while some aromatherapists advocate ingesting small amounts of these oils, this book does not. Consumption of these oils is not necessary for you to receive their full benefits.

BLENDING

In many instances, you'll find only one oil is required for you to meet a specific need or combat an ailment. There may also be occasions, however, in which blending several oils together will offer a more complete range of benefits and help you address a wide spectrum of desires. You can blend oils on your own or purchase readymade blends. Blending is easy and fun. Use your intuition when picking out oils. Experiment freely, using different oils in different amounts to attain different effects. Try blending with three oils first and see how that goes. In most cases, three is all you need for a synergistic blend.

Bergamot, geranium, lavender, and the citrus oils blend well with most other oils, but don't feel obliged to include one of these oils in a blend. Some of the most beneficial blends may not contain any of these oils.

Scintillating Combinations

When combining essential oils, there are no hard and fast rules. A few drops of this, a few drops of that, a splash of something else, and you're set. There are some blends, however, which address some common concerns.

- **To boost clarity and concentration.** Rosemary, geranium, and basil.

- **To boost energy.** Bergamot, neroli, geranium, and lemon.

- **To ease stress.** Lavender, lemon, chamomile, myrrh, sandalwood, frankincense, ylang-ylang, and cedarwood.

- **To fight colds, cough, or flu.** Eucalyptus, ginger, and rosemary.

- **To lift mood.** Orange, eucalyptus, lavender, and neroli.

- **To relieve muscle or joint pain.** Frankincense, ginger, lavender, peppermint, and rosemary.

The previous examples are just a few useful combinations. Mix together your favorites and make your own personal blends.

ORGANIC OR NOT?

Some people prefer to use certified organic essential oils. Organic essential oils are produced from herbs that are grown without the use of synthetic fertilizers or pesticides, irradiation, genetic engineering, growth hormones, or antibiotics. They're as close to natural as you can get. Some aromatherapists prefer to use organic essential oils because of their high quality and the fact that they're unadulterated, meaning they contain none of the undesirable substances listed above. While nonorganic essential oils labeled 100 percent pure are usually more than adequate for the casual aromatherapist, some prefer only the most natural essential oils available. Whether you choose nonorganic but 100-percent pure essential oils or organic essential oils, you can't go wrong. It's really just a matter of preference.

CARE AND STORAGE

To get the most out of your essential oils, it's important to follow a few care and storage rules. First and foremost, essential oils are extremely sensitive to light, temperature extremes, and oxygen. To protect your oils from light, make sure they are housed in brown- or amber-colored bottles. Always make sure lids are on tight, and store them in a cool, dark place. Refrigeration is an option, but be warned that some oils stored this way will become cloudy, although this cloudiness will not affect their therapeutic properties.

Should you choose to store your oils in the refrigerator, take them out an hour prior to use. When cold, essential oils don't flow as freely, so letting them warm up a bit naturally will make them easier to use.

The normal shelf life of most essential oils is two years, but some may last as long as six years with the proper care. If you've made a blend that includes lotion, cream, or readymade massage oil, note that it will last only as long as the carrier oil (usually around six months). To make your blend last longer, add wheat germ oil. It will act as a preservative and extend its shelf life.

ON YOUR WAY

It is time to curl up in your favorite chair with a cup of herbal tea and get acquainted with the oils. As you read about each one, you'll find yourself drawn to certain oils. These will be the ones you'll want to include in your starter kit.

Your Guide to the Many Uses of Essential Oils

The following reference guide has been designed to allow you to match your problem or need to the applicable essential oils to be used in aromatherapy. As always, before using any essential oil, please refer to its detailed description within this book to be sure you use it appropriately and safely.

USE	ESSENTIAL OIL
Acne	Bergamot, Atlas Cedarwood, Virginian Cedarwood, Geranium, Grapefruit, Helichrysum, Juniper Berry, Lavender, Spike Lavender, Lemongrass, Lime, Neroli, Orange, Palmarosa, Patchouli, Rosemary, Rosewood, Sandalwood, Spearmint, Tangerine, Tea Tree, Thyme, Wintergreen.
After-Sun	Camphor, Helichrysum.
Aging	Frankincense, Myrrh, Neroli, Rosewood. *See also* ARTHRITIS; DRY SKIN; LUMBAGO; MEMORY; WARTS; WRINKLES.
Aggression	Atlas Cedarwood. *See also* ANGER.
Agitation	Atlas Cedarwood. *See also* ANGER; ANXIETY; RESENTMENT; STRESS.
Air Freshener	Atlas Cedarwood, Citronella, Lemon, Lemongrass.
Allergies	Oregano, Cabbage Rose, Damask Rose. *See also* HAY FEVER.
Alopecia	Lavender, Spike Lavender. *See also* HAIR LOSS.
Anemia	Lemon.

USE	ESSENTIAL OIL
Anger	Atlas Cedarwood, Myrrh, Cabbage Rose, Damask Rose. *See also* AGITATION; ANXIETY; NERVOUS TENSION; RESENTMENT; STRESS.
Antibacterial	Basil, Black Pepper, Clove, Blue Gum Eucalyptus, Lemon Eucalyptus, Narrow-Leaved Peppermint Eucalyptus, Helichrysum.
Antiperspirant	Patchouli.
Antiseptic	Carrot Seed, Cassia, Blue Gum Eucalyptus, Lemon Eucalyptus, Narrow-Leaved Peppermint Eucalyptus, Grapefruit, Hyssop, Oregano, Rosemary, Tea Tree.
Antispasmodic	Neroli. *See also* COLITIS.
Antiviral	Basil, Oregano.
Anxiety	Basil, Bergamot, Atlas Cedarwood, Roman Chamomile, Cypress, Hyssop, Juniper Berry, Lavender, Spike Lavender, Marjoram, Neroli, Orange, Patchouli, Cabbage Rose, Damask Rose, Clary Sage, Sandalwood, Tangerine, Vanilla, Vetiver, Ylang-Ylang. *See also* AGITATION; ANGER; RESENTMENT; STRESS.
Apathy	Peppermint.
Aphrodisiac	Geranium, Neroli, Sandalwood, Vetiver, Ylang-Ylang.
Appetite	Bergamot, Hyssop, Juniper Berry, Myrrh, Nutmeg, Oregano, Patchouli, Sage.
Arthritis	Balsam Fir Needle, Basil, Black Pepper, Cassia, Atlas Cedarwood, Virginian Cedarwood, Cinnamon, Clove, Blue Gum Eucalyptus, Lemon Eucalyptus, Narrow-Leaved Peppermint Eucalyptus, Ginger, Grapefruit, Juniper Berry, Lime, Marjoram, Nutmeg, Oregano, Peppermint, Rosemary, Sage, Thyme, Vetiver, Wintergreen. *See also* BACK PAIN; JOINT PAIN; LUMBAGO; RHEUMATISM.
Asthma	Anise Seed, Atlas Cedarwood, Virginian Cedarwood, Clove, Frankincense, Hyssop, Lavender, Spike Lavender, Marjoram, Myrrh, Oregano, Peppermint, Pine Needle, Cabbage Rose, Damask Rose, Rosemary, Spearmint, Tea Tree, Thyme.
Athlete's Foot	Geranium, Lemongrass, Myrrh, Palmarosa, Patchouli, Pine Needle, Tea Tree.

USE	ESSENTIAL OIL
Back Pain	Ginger, Oregano, Peppermint, Rosemary, Clary Sage,Wintergreen. *See also* ARTHRITIS; LUMBAGO; MUSCLE PAIN; MUSCLE SPASMS; MUSCLE SPRAINS.
Bacteria, Airborne	Clove, Blue Gum Eucalyptus, Lemon Eucalyptus, Narrow-Leaved Peppermint Eucalyptus.
Bad Breath	Anise Seed, Bergamot, Clove, Nutmeg, Peppermint.
Bedsores	Frankincense, Myrrh.
Bee Stings	Lavender, Spike Lavender. *See also* WASP STINGS.
Bladder Infections	Sandalwood. *See also* URINARY TRACT HEALTH; URINARY TRACT INFECTIONS.
Bladder Issues	Atlas Cedarwood.
Blemishes	Atlas Cedarwood, Frankincense, Helichrysum, Orange, Tea Tree. *See also* CHICKEN POX; WARTS.
Bloating	Hyssop. *See also* FLUID RETENTION; PMS SYMPTOMS.
Blood Pressure, High	Lemon, Marjoram, Ylang-Ylang.
Blood Pressure, Low	Hyssop, Sage.
Boils	Myrrh, Sandalwood.
Boredom	Orange.
Breath, Shortness of	Frankincense.
Bronchial Issues	Lavender, Spike Lavender.
Bronchitis	Anise Seed, Camphor, Carrot Seed, Atlas Cedarwood, Virginian Cedarwood, Cinnamon, Clove, Cypress, Frankincense, Hyssop, Marjoram, Myrrh, Orange, Oregano, Peppermint, Pine Needle, Sage, Spearmint, Tea Tree, Thyme. *See also* CHILLS; COLDS; FEVER; SNEEZING.
Bruises	Camphor, Helichrysum, Hyssop, Marjoram, Thyme.

USE	ESSENTIAL OIL
Burns, Minor	Clove, Lavender, Spike Lavender, Tea Tree, Thyme.
Carpal Tunnel Syndrome	Oregano.
Cellulite	Atlas Cedarwood, Geranium, Grapefruit, Juniper Berry, Lime, Orange, Oregano, Pine Needle, Rosemary, Tangerine.
Cellulitis	Wintergreen.
Chapped Skin	Carrot Seed, Myrrh, Sandalwood, Tea Tree, Ylang-Ylang. *See also* DRY SKIN.
Chest Infections	Allspice, Clove, Sandalwood.
Chicken Pox	Blue Gum Eucalyptus, Lemon Eucalyptus, Narrow-Leaved Peppermint Eucalyptus, Tea Tree.
Chilblains	Geranium, Marjoram, Tea Tree. *See also* FROSTBITE.
Childbirth	*See* LABOR, CHILDBIRTH; LACTATION; POSTNATAL DEPRESSION.
Chills	Camphor, Cinnamon, Clove, Frankincense, Ginger, Orange, Thyme. *See also* COLDS.
Chronic Fatigue Syndrome	Orange, Oregano. *See also* FATIGUE.
Circulatory Issues	Black Pepper, Cinnamon, Cypress, Frankincense, Geranium, Ginger, Hyssop, Lemon, Neroli, Nutmeg, Peppermint, Cabbage Rose, Damask Rose, Thyme, Ylang-Ylang.
Cleanser, Household	Lemon, Lime.
Cognitive Health	Black Pepper, Clove.
Cold Sores	Geranium, Tea Tree.
Colds	Allspice, Anise Seed, Basil, Bergamot, Camphor, Carrot Seed, Cassia, Atlas Cedarwood, Cinnamon, Clove, Frankincense, Ginger, Helichrysum, Hyssop, Juniper Berry, Lemon, Lime, Marjoram, Myrrh, Orange, Oregano, Palmarosa, Pennyroyal, Peppermint, Pine Needle, Rosemary, Rosewood, Spearmint, Tea Tree, Thyme. *See also* CHILLS; FEVER; SNEEZING.
Colitis	Maroc Chamomile. *See also* ANTISPASMODIC.

USE	ESSENTIAL OIL
Concentration	Basil, Hyssop.
Confidence	Jasmine.
Congestion	Balsam Fir Needle, Black Pepper, Virginian Cedarwood, Blue Gum Eucalyptus, Lemon Eucalyptus, Narrow-Leaved Peppermint Eucalyptus, Frankincense, Ginger, Spike Lavender, Lime, Oregano, Peppermint, Pine Needle, Thyme. *See also* SINUSITIS.
Constipation	Lemon, Marjoram, Orange, Patchouli, Peppermint, Cabbage Rose, Damask Rose, Rosemary, Sage, Tangerine.
Corns	Lemon.
Cough	Allspice, Anise Seed, Camphor, Atlas Cedarwood, Virginian Cedarwood, Cypress, Blue Gum Eucalyptus, Lemon Eucalyptus, Narrow-Leaved Peppermint Eucalyptus, Frankincense, Helichrysum, Hyssop, Jasmine, Spike Lavender, Lemon, Lime, Marjoram, Myrrh, Orange, Peppermint, Pine Needle, Cabbage Rose, Damask Rose, Rosewood, Sage, Sandalwood, Tea Tree, Thyme. *See also* COLDS; WHOOPING COUGH.
Cracked Skin	Tea Tree. *See also* CHAPPED SKIN.
Creativity	Hyssop, Orange.
Cramps, Stomach	*See* STOMACH CRAMPS.
Cuts, Minor	Clove, Hyssop, Lavender, Spike Lavender, Lime, Palmarosa, Pine Needle, Thyme.
Cystitis	Bergamot, Atlas Cedarwood, Virginian Cedarwood, Frankincense, Pine Needle, Sandalwood.
Dandruff	Atlas Cedarwood, Virginian Cedarwood, Geranium, Lemon, Patchouli, Rosemary, Sandalwood, Tea Tree.
Decongestant	*See* CONGESTION.
Deodorant	Lime, Patchouli.
Depression	Basil, Bergamot, Roman Chamomile, Grapefruit, Jasmine, Lavender, Spike Lavender, Lemon, Lime, Neroli, Orange, Cabbage Rose, Damask Rose, Rosemary, Clary Sage, Sandalwood, Vanilla, Ylang-Ylang.

USE	ESSENTIAL OIL
Depression, Postnatal	*See* POSTNATAL DEPRESSION.
Dermatitis	Lavender, Spike Lavender, Patchouli, Spearmint, Thyme.
Diarrhea	Cassia, Cinnamon, Clove, Neroli, Peppermint, Rosemary, Sandalwood, Tangerine.
Digestive Issues	Allspice, Anise Seed, Bergamot, Black Pepper, Carrot Seed, Cinnamon, Citronella, Ginger, Hyssop, Lemon, Marjoram, Myrrh, Nutmeg, Pine Needle, Cabbage Rose, Damask Rose, Clary Sage, and Tangerine. *See also* CONSTIPATION; HEARTBURN; INDIGESTION.
Disinfectant	Grapefruit, Juniper Berry, Lime, Orange.
Dreams	Anise Seed.
Drowsiness	Pine Needle.
Dry Skin	Carrot Seed, Sandalwood, Tea Tree, Ylang-Ylang.
Eczema	Bergamot, Atlas Cedarwood, Virginian Cedarwood, Geranium, Hyssop, Juniper Berry, Lavender, Spike Lavender, Myrrh, Orange, Palmarosa, Patchouli, Pine Needle, Sandalwood, Thyme, Vanilla. *See also* DERMATITIS; PSORIASIS.
Emotional Balance	Hyssop.
Energy, Lack of	Jasmine, Lemon.
Enthusiasm	Rosemary.
Exhaustion, Mental	Clove, Grapefruit, Juniper Berry, Lime, Orange, Peppermint, Spearmint.
Exhaustion, Nervous	Cinnamon, Grapefruit, Pine Needle, Rosemary, Spearmint.
Exhaustion, Physical	Palmarosa, Rosewood, Thyme, Ylang-Ylang.
Fainting Spells	Nutmeg, Peppermint.
Fatigue	Balsam Fir Needle, Basil, Bergamot, Black Pepper, Citronella, Frankincense, Grapefruit, Hyssop, Lemon, Palmarosa, Peppermint, Pine Needle, Rosemary, Spearmint. *See also* ENERGY, LACK OF.

USE	ESSENTIAL OIL
Fear	Orange, Tangerine, Ylang-Ylang.
Fertility	Jasmine.
Fever	Bergamot, Lemon, Lime, Orange, Palmarosa, Rosewood, Spearmint, Tea Tree, Wintergreen. *See also* COLDS; FLU.
Fibromyalgia	Wintergreen.
Flatulence	Anise Seed, Bergamot, Lemongrass, Marjoram, Pennyroyal, Peppermint, Spearmint, Tangerine. *See also* GAS, EXCESS.
Fleas	Citronella, Pennyroyal.
Flu	Anise Seed, Basil, Bergamot, Camphor, Carrot Seed, Cassia, Atlas Cedarwood, Cinnamon, Clove, Frankincense, Ginger, Hyssop, Juniper Berry, Lavender, Spike Lavender, Lemon, Orange, Oregano, Palmarosa, Pennyroyal, Peppermint, Pine Needle, Rosemary, Spearmint, Tea Tree, Thyme.
Fluid Retention	Atlas Cedarwood, Grapefruit, Orange, Patchouli, Rosemary, Sage, Tangerine. *See also* BLOATING.
Food Poisoning, Mild	Ylang-Ylang.
Frigidity	Patchouli, Ylang-Ylang.
Frostbite	Geranium. *See also* CHILBLAINS.
Fungal Infections	Myrrh, Oregano, Palmarosa, Patchouli. *See also* ATHLETE'S FOOT; FUNGUS, SKIN.
Fungus, Skin	Atlas Cedarwood. *See also* ATHLETE'S FOOT; FUNGAL INFECTIONS.
Gas, Excess	Black Pepper, Roman Chamomile. *See also* FLATULENCE.
Gingivitis	Myrrh, Orange. *See also* GUM INFECTIONS; GUMS, SORE; GUMS, SPONGY; TOOTHACHE.
Gout	Juniper Berry, Nutmeg, Pennyroyal, Thyme.
Grief	Marjoram, Cabbage Rose, Damask Rose.
Gum Infections	Peppermint, Thyme. *See also* GINGIVITIS; TOOTHACHE.
Gums, Sore	Spearmint. *See also* GINGIVITIS; GUM INFECTIONS; GUMS, SPONGY; TOOTHACHE.
Gums, Spongy	Myrrh. *See also* GINGIVITIS; GUM INFECTIONS; GUMS, SORE; TOOTHACHE.

USE	ESSENTIAL OIL
Hair Loss	Atlas Cedarwood, Juniper Berry, Ylang-Ylang. *See also* ALOPECIA.
Hair, Oily	Atlas Cedarwood, Lemon, Patchouli, Rosemary.
Hangover	Pine Needle. *See also* HEADACHES; MIGRAINES; NAUSEA.
Hay Fever	Lavender, Spike Lavender, Cabbage Rose, Damask Rose. *See also* SNEEZING.
Headaches	Basil, Maroc Chamomile, Roman Chamomile, Citronella, Geranium, Grapefruit, Juniper Berry, Lavender, Spike Lavender, Lemongrass, Marjoram, Neroli, Oregano, Peppermint, Cabbage Rose, Damask Rose, Rosemary, Rosewood, Spearmint, Thyme, Vetiver, Wintergreen. *See also* MIGRAINES.
Heartbeat, Rapid	Ylang-Ylang.
Heartburn	Sandalwood.
Hemorrhoids	Cypress, Frankincense, Myrrh, Nutmeg.
Herpes	*See* COLD SORES.
Hiccups	Anise Seed, Tangerine.
Hyperactivity	Marjoram, Tangerine.
Hysteria	Neroli.
Immune System Health	Atlas Cedarwood, Juniper Berry, Lemon, Lime, Oregano, Rosewood.
Impotence	Nutmeg, Patchouli, Ylang-Ylang.
Indigestion	Marjoram, Oregano, Peppermint, Sage. *See also* CONSTIPATION; DIGESTIVE ISSUES; HEARTBURN.
Infections	Bergamot, Juniper Berry, Rosewood, Tea Tree. *See also* BLADDER INFECTIONS; CHEST INFECTIONS; GUM INFECTIONS; INTESTINAL INFECTIONS; MOUTH INFECTIONS; THROAT INFECTIONS; URINARY TRACT INFECTIONS.
Insect Bites	Roman Chamomile, Patchouli, Tea Tree, Thyme.
Insomnia	Maroc Chamomile, Roman Chamomile, Juniper Berry, Lavender, Spike Lavender, Marjoram, Neroli, Oregano, Clary Sage, Sandalwood, Tangerine, Thyme, Vanilla, Vetiver, Ylang-Ylang.
Intestinal Disorders	Maroc Chamomile, Pennyroyal, Peppermint, Tangerine.
Intestinal Infections	Cinnamon, Palmarosa, Ylang-Ylang.

USE	ESSENTIAL OIL
Irritability	Maroc Chamomile, Tangerine.
Itching	Vanilla.
Jealousy	Cabbage Rose, Damask Rose.
Jet Lag	Lemongrass.
Joint Pain	Lemon, Orange. *See also* LACTATION; ARTHRITIS; LUMBAGO; RHEUMATISM.
Kidney Issues	Cassia, Atlas Cedarwood, Virginian Cedarwood.
Labor, Childbirth	Frankincense, Jasmine. *See also* LACTATION; POSTNATAL DEPRESSION; STRETCH MARKS.
Lactation	Jasmine.
Laryngitis	Frankincense, Thyme. *See also* SORE THROAT; TONSILLITIS.
Lethargy	Neroli, Orange, Rosewood.
Libido	Cinnamon, Ginger, Jasmine, Nutmeg, Patchouli, Cabbage Rose, Damask Rose, Rosewood, Clary Sage, Vanilla.
Listlessness	Lemon, Lime.
Liver Health	Maroc Chamomile.
Lumbago	Marjoram, Wintergreen. *See also* ARTHRITIS; BACK PAIN.
Lymphatic System Health	Ginger, Oregano.
Meditation	Atlas Cedarwood, Frankincense, Hyssop, Rosewood.
Memory	Rosemary, Sage. *See also* AGING.
Menopause	Maroc Chamomile, Geranium, Neroli, Sage, Clary Sage.
Menstrual Health	Basil, Frankincense, Grapefruit, Hyssop, Juniper Berry, Lavender, Spike Lavender, Oregano, Pennyroyal, Cabbage Rose, Damask Rose, Sage.
Menstrual Pain	Anise Seed, Cinnamon, Jasmine, Marjoram, Oregano, Rosemary.

USE	ESSENTIAL OIL
Migraines	Anise Seed, Basil, Maroc Chamomile, Citronella, Lavender, Spike Lavender, Marjoram, Oregano, Peppermint, Cabbage Rose, Damask Rose, Rosemary, Spearmint. *See also* HEADACHES.
Mood Swings	Geranium, Ginger, Lavender, Spike Lavender.
Mouth Infections	Bergamot, Peppermint. *See also* GUM INFECTIONS; ULCERS, MOUTH.
Mucous, Excess	Geranium. *See also* PHLEGM, EXCESS.
Muscle Aches	Anise Seed, Balsam Fir Needle, Carrot Seed, Marjoram, Thyme, Vetiver, Wintergreen. *See also* BACK PAIN; MUSCLE PAIN; MUSCLE SPASMS; MUSCLE SPRAINS; MUSCLE STIFFNESS.
Muscle Pain	Allspice, Black Pepper, Camphor, Clove, Blue Gum Eucalyptus, Lemon Eucalyptus, Narrow-Leaved Peppermint Eucalyptus, Ginger, Lemongrass, Nutmeg, Orange, Oregano, Peppermint, Rosemary, Sage, Clary Sage, Tangerine, Thyme, Wintergreen. *See also* BACK PAIN; MUSCLE SPASMS; MUSCLE SPRAINS; MUSCLE STIFFNESS.
Muscle Spasms	Basil, Clove, Jasmine. *See also* BACK PAIN, MUSCLE ACHES, MUSCLE PAIN, MUSCLE SPRAINS.
Muscle Sprains	Camphor, Jasmine, Marjoram, Oregano, Thyme. *See also* BACK PAIN, MUSCLE ACHES, MUSCLE PAIN.
Muscle Stiffness	Grapefruit, Marjoram. *See also* BACK PAIN; MUSCLE ACHES, MUSCLE PAIN.
Nail Growth	Lime.
Nail Strength	Lemon.
Nausea	Anise Seed, Cassia, Roman Chamomile, Clove, Peppermint, Cabbage Rose, Damask Rose, Rosewood, Spearmint.
Neck, Stiff	*See* STIFF NECK.
Neck Strain	Clary Sage.
Nervous Exhaustion	*See* EXHAUSTION, NERVOUS.

USE	ESSENTIAL OIL
Nervous Tension	Basil, Bergamot, Atlas Cedarwood, Virginian Cedarwood, Geranium, Hyssop, Jasmine, Juniper Berry, Lavender, Spike Lavender, Marjoram, Nutmeg, Orange, Oregano, Palmarosa, Cabbage Rose, Damask Rose, Rosewood, Clary Sage, Sandalwood.
Neuralgia	Neroli.
Nightmares	Lavender, Spike Lavender.
Nosebleeds	Lemon.
Oily Skin	Atlas Cedarwood, Virginian Cedarwood, Citronella, Cypress, Frankincense, Juniper Berry, Lemon, Lemongrass, Lime, Orange, Patchouli, Rosemary, Tangerine, Thyme, Wintergreen, Ylang-Ylang.
Optimism	Jasmine.
Panic	Neroli, Ylang-Ylang.
Perspiration, Excessive	Citronella, Lemongrass, Patchouli, Pennyroyal.
Phlegm, Excess	Hyssop. *See also* MUCOUS, EXCESS.
PMS Symptoms	Roman Chamomile, Geranium, Lemon, Marjoram, Neroli, Orange, Clary Sage, Tangerine, Vanilla. *See also* BLOATING; HEADACHES; MIGRAINES.
Postnatal Depression	Jasmine, Cabbage Rose, Damask Rose, Ylang-Ylang. *See also* DEPRESSION.
Prayer	Frankincense.
Prostate Issues	Pine Needle.
Psoriasis	Bergamot, Virginian Cedarwood, Lavender, Spike Lavender, Orange, Pine Needle. *See also* DERMATITIS; ECZEMA.

USE	ESSENTIAL OIL
Rashes	Lavender, Spike Lavender, Sandalwood.
Repellent, Feline	Citronella.
Repellent, Insect	Camphor, Atlas Cedarwood, Virginian Cedarwood, Citronella, Blue Gum Eucalyptus, Lemon Eucalyptus, Narrow-Leaved Peppermint Eucalyptus, Lavender, Spike Lavender, Lemon, Lemongrass, Patchouli, Pennyroyal, Rosewood, Sandalwood. *See also* REPELLENT, MOSQUITO.
Repellent, Mosquito	Virginian Cedarwood, Geranium.
Repellent, Rodent	Balsam Fir Needle.
Repellent, Termite	Vetiver.
Resentment	Cabbage Rose, Damask Rose. *See also* ANGER; ANXIETY; NERVOUS TENSION; STRESS.
Respiratory Issues	Balsam Fir Needle, Basil, Atlas Cedarwood, Virginian Cedarwood, Cinnamon, Clove, Cypress, Blue Gum Eucalyptus, Lemon Eucalyptus, Narrow-Leaved Peppermint Eucalyptus, Frankincense, Geranium, Ginger, Hyssop, Jasmine, Lime, Rosemary, Sage, Clary Sage, Spearmint.
Restlessness	Tangerine.
Rheumatism	Anise Seed, Basil, Cassia, Atlas Cedarwood, Virginian Cedarwood, Cinnamon, Clove, Blue Gum Eucalyptus, Lemon Eucalyptus, Narrow-Leaved Peppermint Eucalyptus, Frankincense, Ginger, Grapefruit, Juniper Berry, Lemon, Lime, Marjoram, Myrrh, Nutmeg, Oregano, Pine Needle, Rosemary, Sage, Thyme, Wintergreen. *See also* ARTHRITIS; JOINT PAIN; LUMBAGO.
Runny Nose	Ginger.
Sadness	Tangerine. *See also* DEPRESSION; POSTNATAL DEPRESSION.
Scabies	Lemongrass, Pine Needle.
Scars	Frankincense, Lemon, Neroli, Palmarosa, Cabbage Rose, Damask Rose, Rosewood, Tangerine, Vetiver.
Sciatica	Pine Needle, Wintergreen.
Seasickness	Marjoram.

USE	ESSENTIAL OIL
Seasonal Affective Disorder	Orange.
Self-Confidence	Rosemary.
Shingles	Blue Gum Eucalyptus, Lemon Eucalyptus, Narrow-Leaved Peppermint Eucalyptus, Tea Tree.
Sinusitis	Blue Gum Eucalyptus, Lemon Eucalyptus, Narrow-Leaved Peppermint Eucalyptus, Ginger, Lime, Rosemary, Spearmint, Tea Tree, Thyme. *See also* COLDS; SNEEZING.
Skin Care	Carrot Seed, Maroc Chamomile, Jasmine, Juniper Berry, Lemon, Orange, Palmarosa, Cabbage Rose, Damask Rose, Tangerine.
Skin Inflammation	Roman Chamomile, Helichrysum, Hyssop, Clary Sage, Vanilla. *See also* ACNE; DERMATITIS; ECZEMA; FUNGUS, SKIN; PSORIASIS.
Skin, Loose	Patchouli.
Skin, Oily	*See* OILY SKIN.
Skin, Sensitive	Maroc Chamomile.
Sleeping Aid	*See* DROWSINESS; INSOMNIA.
Smoking Cessation	Black Pepper.
Sneezing	Anise Seed, Cinnamon. *See also* COLDS; NASAL CONGESTION.
Sore Throat	Balsam Fir Needle, Bergamot, Geranium, Ginger, Hyssop, Lime, Myrrh, Pine Needle, Cabbage Rose, Damask Rose, Sandalwood, Thyme, Wintergreen. *See also* LARYNGITIS; THROAT INFECTIONS; TONSILLITIS.
Sores	Frankincense, Myrrh, Pine Needle.
Spleen Health	Maroc Chamomile.
Stamina	Black Pepper.
Stiff Neck	Rosemary.

USE	ESSENTIAL OIL
Stimulant	Black Pepper, Carrot Seed.
Stomach Cramps	Anise Seed, Peppermint. *See also* COLITIS; NAUSEA; SEASICKNESS; UPSET STOMACH.
Stress	Balsam Fir Needle, Basil, Bergamot, Black Pepper, Atlas Cedarwood, Virginian Cedarwood, Cinnamon, Clove, Cypress, Geranium, Grapefruit, Hyssop, Jasmine, Juniper Berry, Lavender, Spike Lavender, Lemon, Lemongrass, Marjoram, Myrrh, Neroli, Orange, Palmarosa, Patchouli, Cabbage Rose, Damask Rose, Rosewood, Clary Sage, Spearmint, Thyme, Ylang-Ylang. *See also* AGITATION; ANGER; ANXIETY; RESENTMENT.
Stretch Marks	Neroli, Tangerine. *See also* LABOR, CHILDBIRTH.
Sunburn	Lavender, Spike Lavender, Peppermint, Tea Tree.
Swelling	Oregano.
Tachycardia	*See* HEARTBEAT, RAPID.
Throat Infections	Blue Gum Eucalyptus, Lemon Eucalyptus, Narrow-Leaved Peppermint Eucalyptus, Lemon. *See also* LARYNGITIS; SORE THROAT; TONSILLITIS.
Throat, Sore	*See* LARYNGITIS; SORE THROAT; THROAT INFECTIONS; TONSILLITIS.
Tired Feet	Peppermint.
Tonsillitis	Bergamot, Geranium, Hyssop, Thyme. *See also* LARYNGITIS; SORE THROAT; THROAT INFECTIONS.
Toothache	Allspice, Clove. *See also* GINGIVITIS; GUM INFECTIONS; GUMS, SORE; GUMS, SPONGY.
Trauma	Sage.
Travel Sickness	Peppermint.
Ulcers, Mouth	Lemon, Myrrh, Orange.
Ulcers, Skin	Atlas Cedarwood, Myrrh.
Upset Stomach	Ylang-Ylang. *See also* COLITIS; NAUSEA; SEASICKNESS; STOMACH CRAMPS.
Urinary Tract Health	Bergamot. *See also* BLADDER INFECTIONS; URINARY TRACT INFECTIONS.

USE	ESSENTIAL OIL
Urinary Tract Infections	Virginian Cedarwood, Frankincense. *See also* BLADDER INFECTIONS; URINARY TRACT HEALTH.
Varicose Veins	Cypress, Lime, Tea Tree.
Vascular Disorders	Cassia.
Vertigo	Anise Seed, Atlas Cedarwood, Peppermint.
Vitality	Jasmine.
Voice Loss	Lemon.
Vomiting	Cabbage Rose, Damask Rose, Spearmint. *See also* NAUSEA.
Warts	Clove, Lemon, Tea Tree, Thyme. *See also* BLEMISHES.
Wasp Stings	Lavender, Spike Lavender. *See also* BEE STINGS.
Whooping Cough	Anise Seed, Hyssop, Tea Tree.
Wounds	Bergamot, Carrot Seed, Roman Chamomile, Frankincense, Helichrysum, Hyssop, Juniper Berry, Lime, Myrrh, Palmarosa, Patchouli, Rosewood. *See also* ULCERS, SKIN.
Wrinkles	Carrot Seed, Helichrysum, Myrrh, Rosewood.

ALLSPICE
Pimenta diocia

Many people think allspice is a combination of several spices and are surprised to discover it's actually just one. That's because allspice has a flavor reminiscent of a blend of cloves, cinnamon, and nutmeg. Due to its unique flavor, allspice is a favorite of bakers everywhere and is used in a variety of dishes. You might find it in breads, pies, cakes, relishes, gravies, preserves, or even ketchup. Although allspice is highly esteemed for its place in the kitchen, it is also a widely used aromatic as well, with a variety of "scentsational" benefits.

THERAPEUTIC USES

Chest infections, colds, cough, digestive issues, muscle pain, and toothache.

ESSENTIAL OIL APPLICATIONS

■ For chest infections, colds, or cough, add 2 to 3 drops to 1 ounce of carrier oil and massage into chest and back. Because allspice can irritate skin if used alone, it's important to dilute it in carrier oil.

■ For digestive issues, add 2 to 3 drops to 1 ounce of carrier oil and massage into abdominal area. May also use 2 to 3 drops in a diffuser.

■ For muscle pain, add 2 to 3 drops to 1 ounce of carrier oil and massage into affected areas.

■ For toothache, place 2 to 3 drops on a cotton swab and apply directly to affected tooth. Take great care not to swallow, as the high concentration of allspice in its essential oil could cause nausea.

MIXES WELL WITH: Geranium, ginger, lavender, myrrh, orange, patchouli, and ylang-ylang.

EXTRACTION METHOD: Steam distillation.

PARTS USED: Leaves and fruit.

SAFETY INFORMATION: Avoid if pregnant or nursing. Should not be used neat—that is using only the oil itself—on skin; always mix with carrier oil, lotion, or cream if using on skin.

FUN FACT

The ardent explorer Christopher Columbus discovered allspice in 1494, but it wasn't until the seventeenth century that it was recognized and used as a spice.

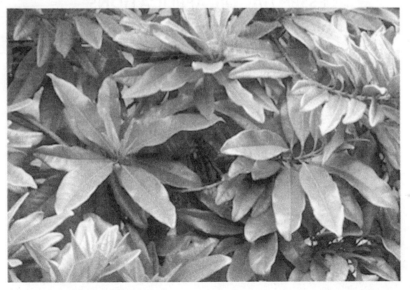

(See color photo on page 76.)

ANISE SEED
Pimpinella anisum

From the sublime to the fantastic, anise seed has been employed in a multitude of ways throughout history. It was used to perfume the clothing of King Edward IV, as a food flavoring during the Middle Ages, and to fund repairs to London Bridge, for which a special tax was added to the sale of anise seed. Pliny the Elder, author of the first encyclopedia, claimed its seeds had the power to prevent bad dreams if placed beneath the sleeper's pillow. Anise seed (or aniseed) is a member of the parsley family, and its flavor resembles licorice. Used medicinally since prehistoric times, anise seed remains a staple in aromatherapy.

THERAPEUTIC USES

Asthma, bad breath, bronchitis, colds, cough, digestive issues, flatulence, flu, hiccups, menstrual pain, migraines, muscle aches, nausea, rheumatism, sneezing, stomach cramps, vertigo, and whooping cough.

ESSENTIAL OIL APPLICATIONS

- For abdominal cramps or severe sneezing, add 5 drops to 1 tablespoon of almond oil and massage into stomach (cramps) or neck (sneezing). Use same mixture for coughs but massage into chest instead.

- For asthma, bronchitis, colds, cough, flu, or whooping cough, use 2 to 3 drops in a steam inhalation. May also be used in a diffuser.

- For bad breath, mix 1 to 2 drops in warm water. Swish and gargle.

- For digestion or hiccups, use 2 to 3 drops in a steam inhalation.

- For menstrual pain or muscle aches, add 2 to 3 drops to 1 ounce of carrier oil and massage into affected areas.

- For migraines or vertigo, use 2 to 3 drops on a handkerchief and inhale periodically. Also useful for digestive issues.

- For nausea, use 2 to 3 drops in a steam inhalation.

MIXES WELL WITH: Cedarwood, lavender, orange, rosewood, clary sage, sandalwood, and tangerine.

EXTRACTION METHOD: Steam distillation.

PARTS USED: Seeds.

SAFETY INFORMATION: Avoid if pregnant or nursing. May cause stomach irritation or dizziness, so do not exceed recommended dosage. Do not use if diagnosed with endometriosis or estrogen-dependent cancer.

FUN FACT

In 1619, it was decreed by law from the Virginia Assembly that each family plant at least six anise seeds a year.

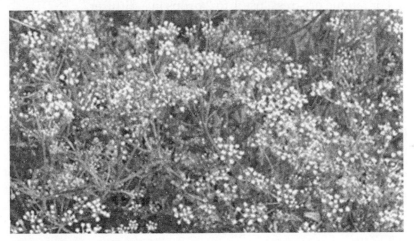

(See color photo on page 76.)

BALSAM FIR NEEDLE
Abies balsamea

The wood and resin of fir trees have been used in a number of ways. The wood has been burned for aromatic and cleansing rituals, while the resin has been applied to wounds to heal and protect them from infection. Fir tree resin is also used to create the solvent known as turpentine. Of course, balsam fir needle oil is derived from steam distillation of balsam fir needles, not resin. It has a pleasant scent that is considered to be balancing and strengthening. It has been known to alleviate congestion due to seasonal illness, and has also been approved as a nontoxic rodent repellent by the Environmental Protection Agency.

THERAPEUTIC USES

Arthritis, fatigue, muscle aches, respiratory issues that accompany the common cold or flu, rodent repellent, sore throat, and stress.

ESSENTIAL OIL APPLICATIONS

■ For arthritis or muscle aches, add 3 to 5 drops to 1 ounce of carrier oil and massage into affected areas.

■ For fatigue or stress, use 1 to 2 drops in a diffuser.

■ For sore throat or respiratory issues, use 1 to 2 drops in a steam inhalation. May also be used in a diffuser.

■ To repel rodents, use a few drops on cotton balls and place in infested areas.

MIXES WELL WITH: Lavender, lemon, marjoram, orange, pine needle, and rosemary.

EXTRACTION METHOD: Steam distillation.

PARTS USED: Needles.

SAFETY INFORMATION: Avoid if pregnant or nursing. May irritate skin, therefore do not use without diluting. Use a patch test before using on skin. Avoid contact with eyes or other mucous membranes.

FUN FACTS

Native Americans have been known to pad their pillows with fir needles to encourage peaceful sleep.

Balsam fir trees are one of the major food supplies for moose in the winter.

The Balsam fir is one of the most popular Christmas trees.

BASIL

Ocimum basilcum

Believed by Hindus to be a passport to heaven, and by one Greek author to exist only to drive men insane, basil enjoys quite the reputation. Of course, basil is most associated with meals, in which it is used as an herb to punch up flavors with its aromatic, mildly pungent qualities. Basil is a favorite among Italian cooks and can be found in a variety of popular dishes. Although many people identify basil with Italy, it is actually native to India and Iran. In India, basil was considered sacred. The name comes from the Greek word "basileus," meaning "king." Currently, there are over 150 varieties of basil, though the variety named *Ocimum basilicum* is most used in aromatherapy.

THERAPEUTIC USES

Antibacterial, antiviral, anxiety, arthritis, colds, concentration, depression, fatigue, flu, headaches, menstrual regulation, migraines, muscle spasms, nervous tension, respiratory issues, rheumatism, and stress.

ESSENTIAL OIL APPLICATIONS

- For antibacterial and antiviral protection, use 2 to 3 drops in a diffuser.

- For anxiety, depression, fatigue, nervous tension, or stress, use 2 to 3 drops in a diffuser. May also add 2 to 3 drops to 1 ounce of carrier oil and massage into body where desired. For added benefit, add lavender or peppermint oil to the mix.

- For arthritis, muscle spasms, or rheumatism, add 2 to 3 drops to 1 ounce of carrier oil and massage into affected areas. May also use in a hot compress.

- For congestion, add 2 to 3 drops to 1 ounce of carrier oil and massage into chest and upper back.

- For headaches or migraines, use 2 to 3 drops in a hot or cold compress (whichever works best for you).

- For respiratory issues, use 2 to 3 drops in a steam inhalation.

- To help regulate menstrual cycle, use 2 to 3 drops in a diffuser regularly.

- To improve concentration, use 2 to 3 drops in a diffuser.

MIXES WELL WITH: Camphor, citronella, citrus oils, clove, eucalyptus, geranium, lavender, myrrh, oregano, peppermint, rosemary, sandalwood, spearmint, and tea tree.

EXTRACTION METHOD: Steam distillation.

PARTS USED: Leaves and flowering tops.

SAFETY INFORMATION: Avoid if pregnant or nursing. May irritate skin, therefore do not use without diluting. Use a patch test before using on skin.

FUN FACT

In Italy, basil is regarded as a sign of love.

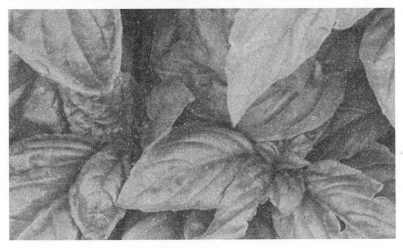

(See color photo on page 76.)

BERGAMOT
Citrus bergamia

The origin of bergamot's name has a rather controversial history. Some say it originated in Northern Italy, with the plant taking its name from the small town of Bergamo, where it was supposedly discovered. Others suggest the name comes from the Turkish word "beg-armande" which means "the king's pear" and reflects the pear-shaped fruit of the plant. Whatever its history, there is no disputing that bergamot has been used for years because of its sweet, citrusy scent with spicy undertones. Popular with perfumers for centuries, bergamot has an uplifting, energizing scent that makes it perfect for aromatherapy. Additionally, bergamot is one of the most versatile essential oils, as it has not only sedative qualities but also stimulating ones. It appears to adapt to the needs of the person using it. Bergamot also gives Earl Grey tea its unmistakable and unique flavor, which makes it a favorite among tea lovers everywhere.

THERAPEUTIC USES

Acne, anxiety, appetite regulation, bad breath, colds, cystitis, depression, digestive issues, eczema, fatigue, fever, flatulence, flu, infections (all types, especially of the skin), nervous tension, psoriasis, sore throat, stress, tonsillitis, urinary tract health, and wounds.

ESSENTIAL OIL APPLICATIONS

■ For acne, eczema, psoriasis, or wounds, add 2 to 3 drops to 1 ounce of jojoba carrier oil and apply directly to affected areas.

■ For anxiety, depression, fatigue, nervous tension, or stress, use 2 to 3 drops in a diffuser.

■ For bad breath, mouth infections, sore throat, or tonsillitis, use 2 to 3 drops in a homemade mouthwash. Gargle and rinse.

- For cystitis or urinary tract health, add 4 to 5 drops to 1 tablespoon of shower gel, shampoo, or Castile soap and mix into bath water for a luxurious, long soak. Also, 2 to 3 drops of bergamot may be added to 1 ounce of carrier oil and massaged into lower abdominal and kidney area to promote optimal health of the excretory system.

- For digestive issues or flatulence, add 2 to 3 drops to 1 ounce of carrier oil and massage into abdominal area. May also use 2 to 3 drops in a diffuser.

- To regulate appetite, use 2 to 3 drops in a diffuser regularly.

MIXES WELL WITH: All essential oils, especially cedarwood, chamomile, citronella, eucalyptus, geranium, juniper berry, lavender, lemon, lime, marjoram, nutmeg, orange, oregano, palmarosa, rosemary, clary sage, sandalwood, tangerine, and ylang-ylang.

EXTRACTION METHOD: Cold expression.

PARTS USED: Peel of nearly ripe fruit.

SAFETY INFORMATION: Avoid if pregnant or nursing. This essential oil is phytotoxic, which means it increases the effects of sunlight. Therefore, never apply bergamot to skin before exposure to sun. Additionally, do not apply neat—that is using only the oil itself—on skin. It must be diluted in carrier oil or cream.

FUN FACT

Bergamot essence is used in voodoo as a protective measure against evil and danger.

BLACK PEPPER
Piper nigrum

Black pepper spice was once one of the most valuable trade items exported from India to the rest of the world. It was even considered sacred. Native to South Asia and Southeast Asia, it is one of the oldest known spices, having been used in Indian cuisine for over 4,000 years. The essential oil of this spice smells like freshly ground peppercorns but does not cause sneezing, which the dried seasoning is known to do. Black pepper essential oil is a stimulant and has been used to improve circulation, encourage proper digestion, relieve muscle aches, and enhance alertness and stamina. Studies have also shown that the inhalation of black pepper essential oil may prove useful to people who are trying to quit smoking, as it seems to alleviate cravings for cigarettes.

THERAPEUTIC USES

Antibacterial, arthritis, circulatory issues, cognitive health, digestive issues, excess gas, fatigue, muscle pain, nasal congestion, smoking cessation, stamina, stimulant, and stress.

ESSENTIAL OIL APPLICATIONS

- For arthritis, circulatory issues, or muscle aches, add 3 to 5 drops to 1 ounce of carrier oil and massage into affected areas.

- For cognitive health, use 2 to 3 drops in a diffuser.

- For digestive issues or excess gas, add 2 to 3 drops to 1 ounce of carrier oil and massage into abdominal area. May also use 2 to 3 drops in a diffuser.

- For fatigue or stress, use 2 to 3 drops in a diffuser.

- For nasal congestion, use 2 to 3 drops in a steam inhalation. May also be used in a diffuser.

To curb cigarette cravings, place a few drops on a cotton ball and smell the aroma.

MIXES WELL WITH: Bergamot, clove, coriander, fennel, frankincense, geranium, ginger, grapefruit, juniper berry, lavender, lemon, lime, sage, clary sage, sandalwood, and ylang-ylang.

EXTRACTION METHOD: Steam distillation.

PARTS USED: Peppercorns.

SAFETY INFORMATION: Avoid if pregnant or nursing. Avoid before bedtime. May irritate skin. Using too much may cause over-stimulation of the kidneys. Do not take internally.

FUN FACTS

Attila the Hun is said to have demanded a ransom of 3,000 pounds of black peppercorns for the city of Rome.

While pepper spice comes in a number of colors, including green, red, black, and white, all variations come from the same plant. The color is related to the ripeness of the plant at the time of processing.

CAMPHOR
Cinnamomum camphora

The unique scent of camphor is most commonly described using two words: powerful and medicinal. Because of its strong aroma, peasants used to wear lumps of camphor around their necks to repel infectious diseases. For over 5,000 years, Ayurvedic medicine has utilized camphor mainly as a germ killer. Camphor was also used in Persia (now Iran) as a remedy for Plague. Even modern-day people turn to camphor to fight cold symptoms. Besides fighting colds, camphor has many other uses. Ancient inhabitants of India used camphor in a variety of religious rituals. The Chinese used camphor wood to build ships and temples, not only for its durability but also for its aromatic properties. Camphor has another unique use as a moth repellent. It's a natural means to protect much-loved wardrobes from the damage moth infestation can cause.

THERAPEUTIC USES

After-sun tonic, bronchitis, bruises, chills, colds, cough, flu, muscle pain, muscle sprains, and insect repellent.

ESSENTIAL OIL APPLICATIONS

■ For bronchitis, colds, cough, or flu, use 2 to 3 drops in a diffuser.

■ For bruises, muscle pain, or muscle sprains, use in a cold compress.

■ Great as an after-sun tonic, but do not use directly on skin. Add 2 drops to 3 tablespoons of liquid lanolin and apply to skin. Do a patch test first to check for sensitivity.

■ To repel insects, use 2 to 3 drops in a diffuser. May also be put on cotton balls and placed in infested areas, but do not place directly on clothes.

MIXES WELL WITH: Basil, chamomile, and lavender.

EXTRACTION METHOD: Steam distillation.

PARTS USED: Wood chips, stumps, and branches.

SAFETY INFORMATION: Camphor is one of the strongest essential oils available, so caution must be exercised when using this particular oil. Avoid if pregnant or nursing, or if diagnosed with epilepsy or asthma. Do not take internally.

FUN FACT
Camphor is used in some cultures
to scare away ghosts.

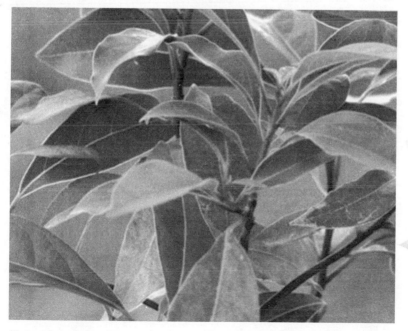

(See color photo on page 76.)

CARROT SEED

Daucus carota

Carrot seed essential oil is appreciated mainly in relation to skin care. It is thought to remove wrinkles and nourish and rejuvenate damaged skin. It is commonly added to facial masks and other preparations for mature skin. It is not appreciated, however, for its aroma, which is rather unpleasant on its own. Thankfully, this scent can be mitigated by mixing carrot seed essential oil with other carrier oils. Carrot seed essential oil is derived from the plant species *Daucus carota*, also known as wild carrot, bird's nest, and bishop's lace. In North America it is called Queen Anne's lace.

THERAPEUTIC USES

Antiseptic, bronchitis, colds, digestive issues, dry or chapped skin, flu, muscle aches, stimulant, wounds, and wrinkles.

ESSENTIAL OIL APPLICATIONS

- For bronchitis, colds, or flu, add 8 to 10 drops to 1 ounce of carrier oil and massage into chest area.

- For digestive issues, add 8 to 10 drops to 1 ounce of carrier oil and massage into abdominal area.

- For dry or chapped skin, wounds, or wrinkles, add 8 to 10 drops to 1 ounce of carrier oil and massage into affected areas.

- For muscle aches or as a stimulant, add 8 to 10 drops to 1 ounce of carrier oil and massage into affected areas.

MIXES WELL WITH: Bergamot, black pepper, cedarwood, cinnamon, cypress, geranium, orange, patchouli, and sandalwood.

EXTRACTION METHOD: Steam distillation.

PARTS USED: Seeds.

SAFETY INFORMATION: Avoid if pregnant or nursing. Do not take internally.

FUN FACTS

Orange-colored carrots appeared in the Netherlands in the seventeenth century. It is thought that the Dutch crossed purple carrot roots with wild carrot types until they arrived at the orange variety.

During World War II, the British circulated a story that RAF gunners, who had been proving themselves quite successful at shooting down German planes at night, had been eating large amounts of carrots to improve their vision. Although carrots certainly encourage healthy eyesight, it was actually new radar technology that had been giving the gunners an edge—a fact the British wished to hide from the Germans.

CASSIA
Cinnamomum cassia

Cassia, also known as Chinese cinnamon, is somewhat similar to cinnamon (*Cinnamomum zeylanicum*) in both taste and therapeutic properties. Although the United States Pharmacopoeia recognizes it as cinnamon, it should not be confused as such, for it has its own unique benefits and history. It has been used for centuries both in medicine and cooking. Germans and Romans preferred to use cassia instead of cinnamon in chocolate, as it has a stronger flavor. Both Europeans and Chinese used cassia in a variety of ways to spice up foods. The Chinese also used cassia frequently for digestive complaints such as diarrhea or nausea. It has also been employed to fight colds, rheumatism, kidney problems, and most particularly vascular disorders. Cassia is also a known skin irritant, so it's best to use it in vapor therapy. Today, cassia is often used in confectionaries and potpourri.

THERAPEUTIC USES

Antiseptic, arthritis, colds, diarrhea, germicide, kidney issues, nausea, rheumatism, and vascular disorders.

ESSENTIAL OIL APPLICATIONS

- As a powerful antiseptic, cassia oil may be mixed with water and sprayed in a sickroom. Add 10 drops to 1 quart of water and pour into a spray bottle. Shake well before spraying.

- For arthritis, colds, diarrhea, kidney issues, nausea, rheumatism, or vascular disorders, use 2 to 3 drops in a diffuser.

MIXES WELL WITH: Cassia is best used on its own.

EXTRACTION METHOD: Steam or water distillation.

PARTS USED: Leaves (steam), or bark, leaves, twigs, and stalks (water).

SAFETY INFORMATION: Avoid if pregnant or nursing. Very large doses can cause depression.

FUN FACT

In the Middle Ages, Europeans used dried cassia buds in Hippocras, a spiced wine.

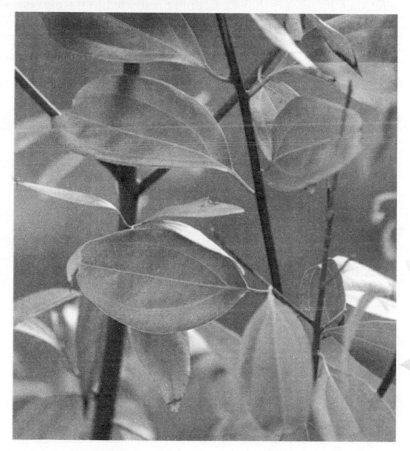

(See color photo on page 76.)

ATLAS CEDARWOOD
Cedrus atlantica

The use of cedarwood oil can be traced back to Biblical times. The Atlas cedar is related to the well-known centuries-old biblical cedars of Lebanon. Today those trees are protected by law from being felled, but the constituents of Atlas cedarwood oil are very much like its ancestors and provide many of the same therapeutic benefits. Warm, sweet, rich, and woody, Atlas cedarwood oil is used in many perfumes and soaps. It produces a calm, meditative state of mind and has the ability to relieve nervous tension, anger, and stress. When used in a diffuser, Atlas cedarwood oil creates a relaxing, quiet atmosphere, perfect for meditating or reflecting. Its powers, however, aren't restricted to the nervous system. Atlas cedarwood oil also works wonders on respiratory and immune systems, and is great for skin. Tibetan traditional medicine still uses it to treat a variety of ailments.

THERAPEUTIC USES

Acne, aggression, agitation, air freshener, anger, anxiety, arthritis, asthma, bladder issues, blemishes, bronchitis, cellulite, colds, cough, cystitis, dandruff, eczema, fluid retention, hair loss, immune system health, insect repellent, kidney issues, meditation, nervous tension, oily hair, oily skin, rheumatism, skin fungus, skin ulcers, stress, and vertigo.

ESSENTIAL OIL APPLICATIONS

▦ As an air freshener, use 2 to 3 drops in a diffuser.

▦ For acne, blemishes, eczema, oily skin, skin fungus, or skin ulcers, add 2 to 3 drops to 1 ounce of carrier oil and dab on affected areas.

▦ For aggression, agitation, anger, anxiety, nervous tension, or vertigo, use 2 to 3 drops in a diffuser.

▦ For arthritis or rheumatism, add 2 to 3 drops to 1 ounce of carrier oil and massage into affected areas. May also add 8 to 10 drops to 1 tablespoon of shower gel, shampoo, or Castile soap and mix into bath water.

- For asthma, bronchitis, colds, or cough, use 2 to 3 drops in a steam inhalation.

- For bladder issues, cystitis, or kidney issues, add 8 to 10 drops to 1 tablespoon of shower gel, shampoo, or Castile soap and mix into bath water.

- For cellulite or fluid retention, add 2 to 3 drops to 1 ounce of carrier oil and massage into affected areas. May also add 8 to 10 drops to 1 tablespoon of shower gel, shampoo, or Castile soap and mix into bath water.

- For dandruff or oily scalp, mix 2 to 3 drops with unscented hair conditioner and massage into scalp. Leave on for 3 to 5 minutes and then rinse.

- For hair loss, add 2 to 3 drops to 1 ounce of carrier oil and massage into scalp periodically.

- To boost the immune system, add 8 to 10 drops to 1 tablespoon of shower gel, shampoo, or Castile soap and mix into bath water, or use 2 to 3 drops in a diffuser.

- To keep meditation focused, put 2 to 3 drops in a diffuser during meditation.

- To repel insects, put a few drops on cotton balls and place in infested areas. Great for ants and moths but also effective against other insects.

MIXES WELL WITH: Bergamot, ginger, juniper berry, marjoram, oregano, patchouli, pine needle, rosemary, rosewood, clary sage, and ylang-ylang.

EXTRACTION METHOD: Steam distillation.

PARTS USED: Wood, stumps, and sawdust.

SAFETY INFORMATION: Avoid if pregnant or nursing. Do not use if diagnosed with high blood pressure or heart problems. Possible irritant to skin. Because scent is stimulating, it may counteract the sedative effects of drugs like pentobarbital. Do not use for more than a few days at a time.

(See color photo on page 76.)

VIRGINIAN CEDARWOOD

Juniperus virginiana

If the smell of a newly sharpened pencil brings back good memories, you'll love the mild, sweet, woody scent of cedarwood. Native Americans valued cedarwood for its healing and purification properties. They used it to combat respiratory infections and treat arthritis. Cedarwood was also used in some ceremonies for purification. Egyptians also valued cedarwood and used it in the mummification process, in cosmetics, and to repel insects. Insects and rats hate the smell of cedarwood, so it makes a great repellent, especially against mosquitoes, moths, and woodworms. In fact, at one time cedarwood was combined with citronella and used as a commercial insecticide. Today, aromatherapists use cedarwood in a variety of capacities, from insect repellent to mood relaxer.

THERAPEUTIC USES

Acne, arthritis, asthma, bronchitis, congestion, cough, cystitis, dandruff, eczema, insect repellent, kidney issues, nervous tension, oily skin, psoriasis, rheumatism, stress, and urinary tract infections.

ESSENTIAL OIL APPLICATIONS

- For acne, eczema, psoriasis, or oily skin, add 2 to 3 drops to 1 ounce of carrier oil and dab on affected areas.

- For arthritis or rheumatism, add 2 to 3 drops to 1 ounce of carrier oil and massage into affected areas. May also add 8 to 10 drops to 1 tablespoon of shower gel, shampoo, or Castile soap and mix into bath water.

- For asthma, bronchitis, congestion, or cough, use 2 to 3 drops in a steam inhalation.

- For cystitis, kidney issues, or urinary tract infections, add 8 to 10 drops to 1 tablespoon of shower gel, shampoo, or Castile soap and mix into bath water.

- For dandruff, mix 2 to 3 drops with unscented hair conditioner and massage into scalp. Leave on for 3 to 5 minutes and then rinse.

- To alleviate nervous tension or stress, use 2 to 3 drops in a diffuser.

- To repel insects or rats, put a few drops on cotton balls and place in infested areas. May also use 2 to 3 drops in a diffuser.

MIXES WELL WITH: Anise seed, bergamot, chamomile, citronella, eucalyptus, ginger, juniper berry, lavender, lemon, palmarosa, patchouli, pine needle, rosemary, and sandalwood.

EXTRACTION METHOD: Steam distillation.

PARTS USED: Wood chips and sawdust.

SAFETY INFORMATION: Avoid if pregnant or nursing. May irritate skin. Do a patch test first.

FUN FACT

Cedarwood is used to make pencils, which makes its aroma reminiscent of school days gone by.

(See color photo on page 77.)

MAROC CHAMOMILE

Ormenis multicaulis

Chamomile is the great relaxer. It's been used for centuries to calm and soothe mind, body, and soul. In fact, in the language of flowers its name means "patience in adversity." Maroc chamomile (*Ormenis multicaulis*) should not be confused with German or Roman chamomile, as it is not derived from a true chamomile plant. It also has its own set of unique benefits. This particular essential oil is good for ailments such as sensitive skin, colitis, headaches and migraines, irritability, insomnia, and menopause. While effective on its own, chamomile can help boost the power of lavender and cedarwood essential oils.

THERAPEUTIC USES

Colitis, headaches, insomnia, intestinal disorders, irritability, liver or spleen congestion, menopause, migraines, and sensitive skin.

ESSENTIAL OIL APPLICATIONS

- For colitis, intestinal disorders, or liver or spleen congestion, add 5 to 8 drops to 1 ounce of carrier oil and massage into body. May also add 8 to 10 drops to 1 tablespoon of shower gel, shampoo, or Castile soap and mix into bath water, or use a few drops in a diffuser.

- For headaches or migraines, use 2 to 3 drops in a hot or cold compress (whichever works best for you).

- For insomnia, use 5 to 6 drops in a diffuser. May also place 2 to 3 drops on a tissue and place the tissue inside your pillow before bedtime. Replace nightly. For added benefit, add lavender to the mix.

- For sensitive skin, dilute 1 drop of chamomile with 1 teaspoon of carrier oil such as sweet almond and dab on skin.

- For symptoms of menopause, add 8 drops to 1 ounce of carrier oil and massage into body regularly. May also use a few drops in a diffuser nightly or add 8 to 10 drops to 1 tablespoon of shower gel, shampoo, or Castile soap and mix into bath water.

MIXES WELL WITH: Cedarwood and lavender.

EXTRACTION METHOD: Steam distillation.

PARTS USED: Flowering tops.

SAFETY INFORMATION: Avoid if pregnant or nursing. Avoid if asthmatic.

FUN FACTS

Although Roman chamomile essential oil is light blue to yellow in color, Maroc chamomile is yellow to brown.

❧

The therapeutic use of Maroc chamomile is a relatively recent occurrence, while the use of Roman chamomile dates back to ancient Egypt.

ROMAN CHAMOMILE
Chamaemelum nobile

Chamomile has been used as an herbal remedy since ancient times. The word "chamomile" comes from the Greek words "khamai," meaning on the ground (roman chamomile grows low to the ground), and "melon," meaning apple (roman chamomile has an appealing fruity aroma). This plant has parsley-like leaves and daisy-like flowers, the latter of which are distilled to create its essential oil. Roman chamomile also has the nickname "the plant's physician," as it tends to have positive effects on plants growing nearby. The most common use of chamomile is in teas, but roman chamomile may also be used in face creams, shampoos, and perfumes. It is known to be calming.

THERAPEUTIC USES

Anxiety, depression, excess gas, headaches, insect bites, insomnia, nausea, PMS symptoms, skin inflammation, and wounds.

ESSENTIAL OIL APPLICATIONS

- For excess gas, add 5 to 8 drops to 1 ounce of carrier oil and massage into lower abdominal area. May also add 8 to 10 drops to 1 tablespoon of shower gel, shampoo, or Castile soap and mix into bath water, or use a few drops in a diffuser.

- For headaches, use 2 to 3 drops in a hot or cold compress (whichever works best for you).

- For insomnia, use 5 to 6 drops in a diffuser. May also place 2 to 3 drops on a tissue and place the tissue inside your pillow before bedtime. Replace nightly. For added benefit, add lavender to the mix.

- For skin inflammation, dilute 1 drop of chamomile with 1 teaspoon of carrier oil and dab on skin.

- For PMS symptoms, add 8 drops to 1 ounce of carrier oil and massage into body regularly. May also use a few drops in a diffuser nightly, or add 8 to 10 drops to 1 tablespoon of shower gel, shampoo, or Castile soap and mix into bath water.

MIXES WELL WITH: Bergamot, eucalyptus, geranium, grapefruit, jasmine, lavender, lemon, neroli, palmarosa, rose, clary sage, and tea tree.

EXTRACTION METHOD: Steam distillation.

PARTS USED: Flowering tops.

SAFETY INFORMATION: Avoid if pregnant or nursing. Avoid if asthmatic. May irritate skin.

FUN FACTS

Ancient Romans used this oil
for courage during war.

Before chemical hair dye became widely
available, chamomile was traditionally
used to lighten hair.

(See color photo on page 77.)

CINNAMON
Cinnamomum zeylanicum

The smell of cinnamon wafting through the kitchen is one the most beloved aromas in history. First mentioned in Chinese literature as early as 2700 BC, cinnamon is considered a "warm" herb and is valued in many ancient traditional medical systems, including Ayurvedic medicine. Early Europeans considered cinnamon a "rare and precious spice," and it was often used in tonics to treat a variety of ailments. Used in just about every kitchen of every culture, cinnamon is treasured for its culinary magic as well as its therapeutic benefits. The kitchen and the doctor's office, however, aren't the only places this delicious spice shines. It is also highly valued in the world of aromatherapy for its warming and comforting qualities. Cinnamon oil is especially good for colds, flu, arthritis, rheumatism, and other aches and pains. It also blends well with other oils, especially citrus and spice scents. Cinnamon oil is also great to use in a diffuser before parties or open houses, as it lends a homey, welcoming quality that people find appealing.

THERAPEUTIC USES

Arthritis, bronchitis, chills, circulatory issues, colds, diarrhea, digestive issues, flu, intestinal infections, libido, menstrual pain, nervous exhaustion, rheumatism, sneezing, and stress.

ESSENTIAL OIL APPLICATIONS

- Because cinnamon oil should never be used in a bath or neat—that is using only the oil itself—on skin, vapor therapy is most recommended for the above-referenced ailments. Use 2 to 5 drops in a diffuser. For severe respiratory conditions, such as acute bronchitis, steam inhalation is also a viable alternative. May also add 3 to 4 drops to 1 ounce of carrier oil and massage into body, although this is not recommended for those with sensitive skin.

MIXES WELL WITH: Bergamot, clove, frankincense, geranium, ginger, grapefruit, lavender, lemon, marjoram, nutmeg, orange, patchouli, rose, rosemary, tangerine, thyme, and ylang-ylang.

EXTRACTION METHOD: Steam distillation.

PARTS USED: Leaves and twigs (dried inner bark).

SAFETY INFORMATION: Avoid if pregnant or nursing. Not to be used if under the age of eighteen. People with sensitive skin should avoid cinnamon completely. Do not use in baths. May irritate mucous membranes, so use with care.

FUN FACTS

Cinnamon was once so highly valued that it was used as a trade commodity between India, China, and Egypt.

Roman Emperor Nero burned a year's supply of cinnamon at the funeral of his wife as a display of remorse for having killed her.

CITRONELLA
Cymbopogon winterianus

Citronella is a scent everyone knows but might not love. Used for centuries mainly as an insect repellent, citronella actually has a wide variety of other uses. Look closely and you'll find it as an ingredient in many perfumes, soaps, skin lotions, and deodorants. Citronella is a versatile essential oil, and is a must for anyone who lives in a hot, humid environment.

THERAPEUTIC USES

Digestive issues, excessive perspiration, fatigue, feline repellent, fleas, headaches, insect repellent, migraines, oily skin, and sickroom air freshener.

ESSENTIAL OIL APPLICATIONS

- For digestive issues, add 2 drops to 2 to 3 tablespoons of carrier oil and massage into abdominal area.

- For dogs with fleas, add a couple of drops to a "doggie bandana" or an absorbent collar such as woven nylon and place around dog's neck. Do not use this method for cats, as felines are much more sensitive to this scent.

- For excessive perspiration, add 2 to 3 drops to 1 ounce of carrier oil and apply to armpits.

- For headaches or migraines, use 2 to 3 drops in a cold or hot compress.

- For oily skin, add 2 to 3 drops to 1 ounce of carrier oil and dab on face with a cotton ball.

- For those who are bedridden, citronella is a great freshener for a sickroom. Place a couple of drops in a diffuser. Will also help to clear the mind at the same time.

- To keep neighborhood cats from digging up your garden, mix 10 to 12 drops of oil in a plastic spray bottle full of water and spray around your garden. Do not spray directly on plants.

- To repel insects, use a few drops in a diffuser. Works especially well if used by an open window. Be careful if used indoors, as it can adversely affect caged birds.

- To repel moths, put a few drops on cotton balls and place in infested areas. Refresh periodically.

MIXES WELL WITH: Basil, bergamot, cedarwood, eucalyptus, geranium, lavender, lemon, lime, oregano, pennyroyal, pine needle, rosemary, orange, and tea tree.

EXTRACTION METHOD: Steam distillation.

PARTS USED: Fresh, part-dried, or dried grass.

SAFETY INFORMATION: Avoid if pregnant or nursing.

FUN FACT
Citronella has been used in exorcism rituals to get rid of demons.

(See color photo on page 77.)

CLOVE

Eugenia caryophyllata

Cloves were important in the earliest spice trades, probably because of their prominent role in flavoring foods. Known for their hot, spicy, pungent flavor, cloves are a favorite seasoning spice for meats, baked goods, and beverages. Besides its beloved place in the kitchen, clove essential oil is a valued aromatic and used traditionally as a remedy for skin conditions, to calm digestive upset, and to relieve nausea. It's best known, however, for its use as both a breath freshener and toothache reliever. Cloves remain an important spice commodity, and today are used in everything from perfume to mulled wines, and from love potions to pomades.

THERAPEUTIC USES

Antibacterial, arthritis, asthma, bad breath, bronchitis, burns, chest infections, chills, cognitive function, colds, cuts, diarrhea, mental exhaustion, flu, muscle pain, muscle spasms, nausea, rheumatism, stress, toothache, and warts.

ESSENTIAL OIL APPLICATIONS

- For arthritis, muscle spasms, or rheumatism, add 1 drop to 1 ounce of carrier oil and massage into affected areas.

- For asthma, bronchitis, chest infections, or other respiratory problems, use 2 to 3 drops in a steam inhalation. May also use a few drops in a diffuser.

- For bad breath, dilute in water or clear alcohol (1-percent clove oil). Swish in mouth, spit out, and then rinse mouth with water.

- For burns, cuts, or warts, add 2 to 3 drops to 1 ounce of carrier oil and dab on affected areas.

- For chills, colds, or flu, add 2 to 3 drops to 1 ounce of carrier oil and massage into chest.

- For diarrhea, add 2 to 3 drops in 1 ounce of carrier oil and massage into lower back and abdominal area.

- For mental exhaustion, stress, or cognitive health, use 2 to 3 drops in a diffuser. May also add 2 to 3 drops to 1 ounce of carrier oil and massage into body.

- For toothache, put 2 to 3 drops on a cotton swab and place directly on tooth. May also add 1 drop to 1 ounce of carrier oil and massage into jawline.

- To fight airborne bacteria, use 2 to 3 drops in a diffuser.

MIXES WELL WITH: Cinnamon, geranium, ginger, grapefruit, jasmine, lavender, lemon, myrrh, nutmeg, orange, palmarosa, rose, clary sage, sandalwood, tangerine, tea tree, and ylang-ylang.

EXTRACTION METHOD: Steam distillation.

PARTS USED: Sun-dried buds.

SAFETY INFORMATION: Avoid if pregnant or nursing. May irritate skin, so make sure to dilute clove essential oil with carrier oil, cream, or lotion. May irritate mucous membranes, so when using a vaporizer or a diffuser, be sure to limit exposure. Do not use on a tooth that is currently being worked on by a dentist for root canal. Do not use in baths.

FUN FACT

During the Han Dynasty, cloves were known as "tongue spice" and courtiers were required to hold cloves in their mouths when talking to the emperor.

(See color photo on page 77.)

CYPRESS
Cupressus sempervirens

In ancient times, cypress was known as the tree that lives forever. In modern times, its ability to resist forest fires has brought attention to this tree. Cypress trees hold religious significance in many cultures. In Tibetan culture, it is often used to make incense. It is known to have a refreshing effect on the mind, dispelling worry and stress in those who smell its scent. The astringent properties of this essential oil make it a good treatment for oily or sweaty skin, and its circulatory benefits have been put to use against varicose veins and broken capillaries. Cypress essential oil is also used to aid in respiratory health and to ease stress and anxiety.

THERAPEUTIC USES

Anxiety, bronchitis, circulatory issues, cough, hemorrhoids, oily skin, stress, varicose veins.

ESSENTIAL OIL APPLICATIONS

- For anxiety or stress, use 5 drops in a diffuser. May also add 2 to 3 drops to 1 ounce of carrier oil and massage into body.

- For bronchitis or cough, use 2 to 3 drops in a steam inhalation. May also use a few drops in a diffuser.

- For hemorrhoids or varicose veins, add 5 drops to 1 ounce of carrier oil and massage into affected areas.

- For oily skin, add 1 to 3 drops to 1 ounce of carrier oil and massage on affected areas.

MIXES WELL WITH: Bergamot, black pepper, cedarwood, chamomile, citrus oils, ginger, lavender, pine needle, clary sage, and ylang-ylang.

EXTRACTION METHOD: Steam distillation.

PARTS USED: Needles and Twigs.

SAFETY INFORMATION: Avoid if pregnant or nursing. Keep out of eyes, ears, and nose.

FUN FACT

Cypress trees are associated with death and the afterlife. They are often planted in graveyards and cypress wood may be used to make coffins.

Cypress trees have "knees," which are actually growths that sprout around the tree at a height of several feet from the base. They are thought to increase the oxygen supply to submerged roots.

BLUE GUM EUCALYPTUS
Eucalyptus globulus

Centuries ago, the eucalyptus tree was thought to cleanse the environment, so the frail and sickly would choose to live in areas where these fragrant trees grew, hoping for recovery from their ailments. While just living under the trees might not be the cure people hoped for, the tree does indeed offer healing. The Australian Aborigines applied crushed eucalyptus leaves to wounds to promote healing. They also used eucalyptus leaves to fight infections and relieve muscular pain. In India, eucalyptus is used to cool fever and fight contagious diseases. Even Western surgeons recognized the benefits of eucalyptus and have used a eucalyptus solution to wash out operation cavities. Today, eucalyptus is used in many different types of pharmaceutical products, from vapor rubs to cold remedies. Even veterinarians and dentists use eucalyptus in their practices. Its sweet, menthol, woody scent coupled with its proven healing abilities makes it a favorite essential oil in aromatherapy.

THERAPEUTIC USES

Antibacterial, antiseptic, arthritis, chicken pox, cough, decongestant, insect repellent, muscle pain, rheumatism, shingles, sinusitis, and throat infections.

ESSENTIAL OIL APPLICATIONS

- For arthritis, muscle pain, or rheumatism, add 2 to 3 drops to 1 ounce of carrier oil and massage into affected areas.

- For chicken pox or shingles, use 2 to 3 drops on a cotton swab and apply to affected areas. Relieves pain associated with these ailments.

- For cough, sinusitis, stuffed up noses, or throat infections, use 5 to 7 drops in a diffuser. May also be mixed in carrier oil and massaged into chest.

- To freshen up garbage bins, place a few drops on a paper towel and wipe over lid or place at the bottom of the bin to kill germs and smells.

- To guard against fly infestation, put a few drops on ribbon and hang ribbon near windows or place on windowsills. Refresh weekly.

- To kill airborne bacteria in a sickroom, add 10 drops to 1 quart of water and pour into a spray bottle. Shake well before spraying.

- To repel insects, mix with bergamot and lavender in equal amounts. If applying to skin, use with carrier oil. If using in a linen closet, apply to cotton balls and place on shelves.

MIXES WELL WITH: Basil, bergamot, cedarwood, citronella, ginger, grapefruit, juniper berry, lavender, lemon, lime, marjoram, orange, oregano, peppermint, pine needle, rosemary, spearmint, tea tree, and thyme.

EXTRACTION METHOD: Steam distillation.

PARTS USED: Fresh or partially dried leaves and young twigs.

SAFETY INFORMATION: Avoid if pregnant or nursing. Keep away from babies and small children. Do not use if diagnosed with high blood pressure or epilepsy. Always use in dilution. Do not take internally. Avoid if taking homeopathic remedies, as eucalyptus may act as an antidote to such therapies. May cause topical skin irritation or complications for people with certain medical conditions or prescriptions.

(See color photo on page 77.)

LEMON EUCALYPTUS

Eucalyptus citriodora

Lemon eucalyptus has many of the same therapeutic qualities as the other eucalyptus species mentioned earlier but also has a pleasant lemony scent. Lemon eucalyptus essential oil is known to treat respiratory infections, repel disease-bearing insects, relieve muscle pain, and soothe inflammation, among other uses. While most research on lemon eucalyptus oil focuses on its use as insect repellent, traditional Chinese and Indian systems of medicine have used lemon eucalyptus extract to treat many health conditions, from congestion and coughs to rheumatism. The lemon eucalyptus plant is native to northern Australia and is a tall tree that can reach over 150-feet in height.

THERAPEUTIC USES

Antibacterial, antiseptic, arthritis, chicken pox, cough, decongestant, insect repellent, muscle pain, rheumatism, shingles, sinusitis, and throat infections.

ESSENTIAL OIL APPLICATIONS

- For arthritis, muscle pain, or rheumatism, add 2 to 3 drops to 1 ounce of carrier oil and massage into affected areas.

- For chicken pox and shingles, place 2 to 3 drops on a cotton swab and apply to affected areas. Relieves pain associated with these ailments.

- For cough, sinusitis, stuffed up noses, or throat infections, use 5 to 7 drops in a diffuser. May also be mixed in carrier oil and massaged into chest.

- To freshen up garbage bins, place a few drops on a paper towel and wipe over lid or place at the bottom of the bin to kill germs and smells.

- To guard against fly infestation, put a few drops on ribbon and hang ribbon near windows or place on windowsills. Refresh weekly.

- To kill airborne bacteria in a sickroom, add 10 drops to 1 quart of water and pour into a spray bottle. Shake well before spraying.

- To repel insects, mix equal amounts with bergamot and lavender. If applying to skin, use in carrier oil. If using in a linen closet, apply to cotton balls and place on shelves.

MIXES WELL WITH: Basil, bergamot, cedarwood, citronella, ginger, grapefruit, juniper berry, lavender, lemon, lime, marjoram, orange, oregano, peppermint, pine needle, rosemary, spearmint, tea tree, and thyme.

EXTRACTION METHOD: Steam distillation.

PARTS USED: Fresh or partially dried leaves and young twigs.

SAFETY INFORMATION: Avoid if pregnant or nursing. Keep away from babies and small children. Do not use if diagnosed with high blood pressure or epilepsy. Always use in dilution. Do not take internally. Avoid if taking homeopathic remedies, as eucalyptus acts as an antidote to such therapies. May cause topical skin irritation or complications for people with certain medical conditions or prescriptions.

FUN FACT

Eucalyptus leaves have been used for thousands of years in traditional Aboriginal bush medicine.

NARROW-LEAVED PEPPERMINT EUCALYPTUS
Eucalyptus radiata

Narrow-leaved peppermint, or *Eucalyptus radiata*, is known for its cool, crisp fragrance, which makes it helpful for clear breathing. It is rich in a compound called cineole, which gives it its spicy, cooling scent. *Eucalyptus radiata* essential oil is typically seen as a mild form of eucalyptus oil, as it has a softer aroma than *Eucalyptus globulus,* although it has many of the same properties as this latter type of oil and is often combined with it to promote a healthy respiratory system. Narrow-leaved peppermint eucalyptus essential oil is also considered the most therapeutically versatile of all eucalyptus oils.

THERAPEUTIC USES

Antibacterial, antiseptic, arthritis, chicken pox, cough, decongestant, insect repellent, muscle pain, rheumatism, shingles, sinusitis, and throat infections.

ESSENTIAL OIL APPLICATIONS

- For chicken pox and shingles, place 2 to 3 drops on a cotton swab and apply to affected areas. Relieves pain associated with these ailments.

- For cough, sinusitis, stuffed up noses, or throat infections, use 5 to 7 drops in a diffuser. May also be mixed in carrier oil and massaged into chest.

- To freshen up garbage bins, place a few drops on a paper towel and wipe over lid or place at the bottom of the bin to kill germs and smells.

- To guard against fly infestation, put a few drops on ribbon and hang ribbon near windows or place on windowsills. Refresh weekly.

- For arthritis, muscle pain, or rheumatism, add 2 to 3 drops to 1 ounce of carrier oil and massage into affected areas.

- To kill airborne bacteria in a sickroom, add 10 drops to 1 quart of water and pour into a spray bottle. Shake well before spraying.

- To repel insects, mix equal amounts with bergamot and lavender. If applying to skin, use in carrier oil. If using in a linen closet, apply to cotton balls and place on shelves.

MIXES WELL WITH: Basil, bergamot, cedarwood, citronella, ginger, grapefruit, juniper berry, lavender, lemon, lime, marjoram, orange, oregano, peppermint, pine needle, rosemary, spearmint, tea tree, and thyme.

EXTRACTION METHOD: Steam distillation.

PARTS USED: Fresh or partially dried leaves and young twigs.

SAFETY INFORMATION: Avoid if pregnant or nursing. Keep away from babies and small children. Do not use if diagnosed with high blood pressure or epilepsy. Always use in dilution. Do not take internally. Avoid if taking homeopathic remedies, as eucalyptus acts as an antidote to such therapies. May cause topical skin irritation or complications for people with certain medical conditions or prescriptions.

FUN FACT

Eucalyptus radiata is one of the smaller varieties of this evergreen species of tree, reaching a maximum height of approximately fifty feet, and is native to southwestern Australia.

FRANKINCENSE

Boswellia carteri

Frankincense was one of the gifts given to the baby Jesus from the three Magi. People often wonder why this is so—after all, isn't it just a nicely scented tree? Actually, at one time, frankincense was valued as highly as gold. It was held in this high regard for thousands of years. Frankincense not only had many healing properties but was also burned to rid the sick of evil spirits and purify body and soul. Because of its ability to slow down and deepen the breath, frankincense helps keep prayer and meditation focused. Unsurprisingly, the Egyptians used it in the embalming process, but they also used it in cosmetic facial masks. Today, frankincense remains highly valued by aromatherapists. Possessing qualities that take care of both external and internal problems, it truly is worth its weight in gold.

THERAPEUTIC USES

Aging skin, asthma, bedsores, blemishes, bronchitis, chills, circulatory issues, colds, cough, cystitis, fatigue, flu, heavy periods, hemorrhoids, labor, laryngitis, meditation, menstrual health, nasal congestion, oily skin, prayer, rheumatism, scars, shortness of breath, sores, urinary tract infections, and wounds.

ESSENTIAL OIL APPLICATIONS

- During labor, use a few drops in a diffuser. It will help calm the mother-to-be and also help her focus, especially if using Lamaze.

- During menstruation, add 8 to 10 drops to 1 tablespoon of shower gel, shampoo, or Castile soap and mix into bath water and take a nice, long soak. Helps with a variety of menstrual issues, like cramps, loss of focus, and fatigue.

- For asthma, bronchitis, cough, colds, flu, or laryngitis, add 2 to 3 drops to 1 ounce of carrier oil. Rub into chest for asthma, bronchitis, cough, or colds, and rub on throat for laryngitis. May also use 2 to 3 drops in a diffuser or steam inhalation.

- For bedsores, scars, or wounds, use 2 to 3 drops in a cold compress and apply to affected areas. May also be added to a cotton ball and dabbed on directly; use lightly.

- For blemishes or oily skin, wet a cotton ball and add 1 or 2 drops of oil. Dab on affected areas lightly.

- For chills or circulatory issues, add 4 to 5 drops to 1 ounce of carrier oil and massage into body. May also add 4 to 5 drops to 1 tablespoon of shower gel, shampoo, or Castile soap and mix into bath water.

- For fatigue, use 3 to 5 drops in a diffuser.

- For heavy periods, add 3 to 4 drops to 1 ounce of carrier oil and massage into lower abdominal area regularly.

- For hemorrhoids, add 2 to 3 drops to 2 tablespoons of liquid lanolin and massage into affected areas.

- For mature complexions, wash face, and then add 2 to 3 drops to 1 ounce of almond carrier oil and rub gently on face.

- For nasal congestion, sprinkle a few drops on a handkerchief and inhale periodically. Or use 2 to 3 drops in a diffuser or steam inhalation.

- For prayer or meditation, use 4 to 5 drops in a diffuser.

- For rheumatism, add 3 to 5 drops to 1 ounce of carrier oil and massage into affected areas. May also use in a hot compress.

- For shortness of breath, use 3 to 5 drops in a steam inhalation or diffuser.

- For urinary tract infections, add 8 to 10 drops to 1 tablespoon of shower gel, shampoo, or Castile soap and mix into bath water in addition to using doctor-prescribed medication.

MIXES WELL WITH: Bergamot, cinnamon, clary sage, geranium, grapefruit, jasmine, lavender, lemon, myrhh, neroli, orange, patchouli, pine needle, rose, sandalwood, tangerine, and ylang-ylang.

EXTRACTION METHOD: Steam distillation.

PARTS USED: Oleoresin.

SAFETY INFORMATION: There are no special precautions for humans, but it is not safe for cats. It is also best to use it in moderation.

(See color photo on page 77.)

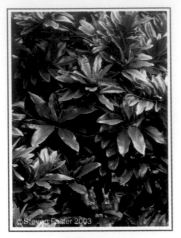

Allspice

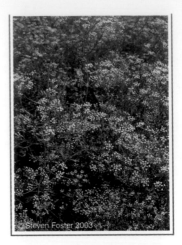

Anise

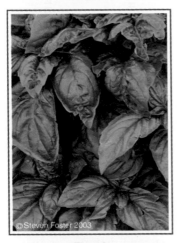

Basil

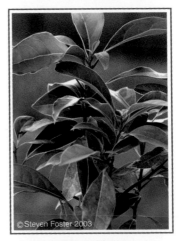

Camphor

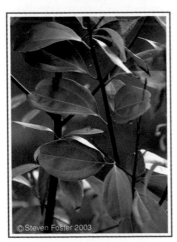

Cassia

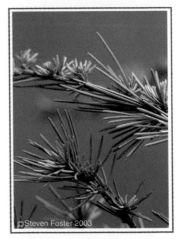

Atlas Cedarwood

76

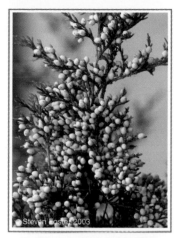

Virginian Cedarwood

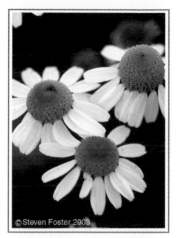

Roman Chamomile

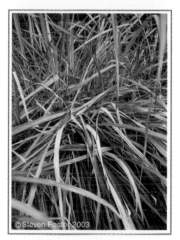

Citronella

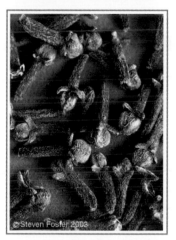

Clove

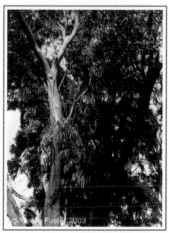

Blue Gum Eucalyptus

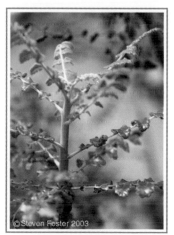

Frankincense

77

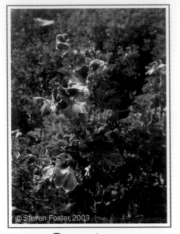

Geranium

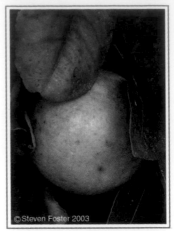

Grapefruit

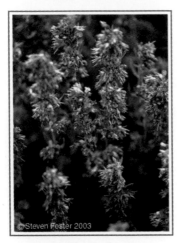

Hyssop

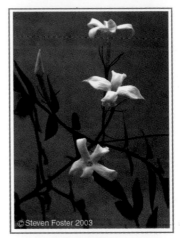

Jasmine

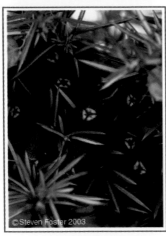

Juniper Berry

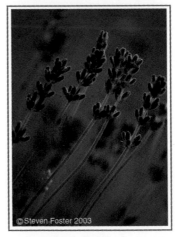

Lavender

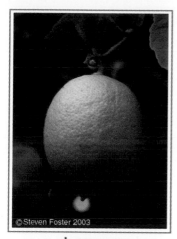

Lemon

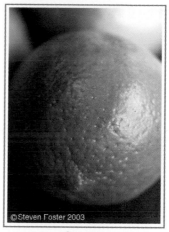

Lime

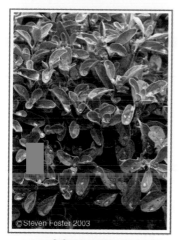

Marjoram

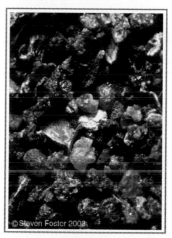

Myrrh

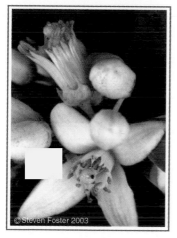

Neroli

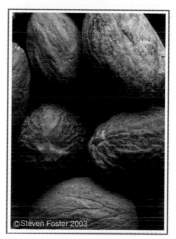

Nutmeg

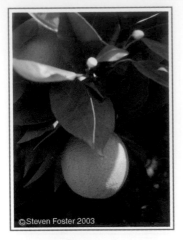

Orange

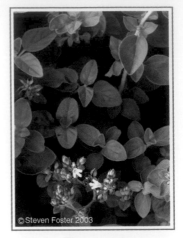

Oregano

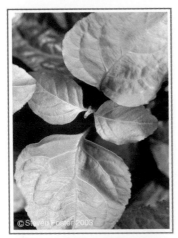

Patchouli

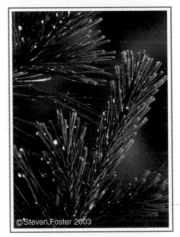

Pine Needle

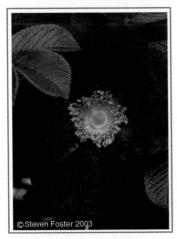

Damask Rose

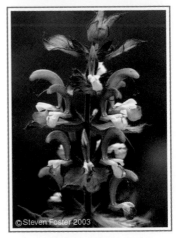

Clary Sage

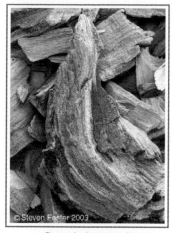

Sandalwood

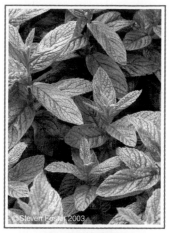

Spearmint

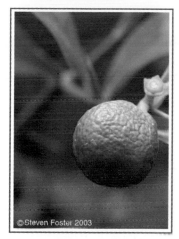

Tangerine

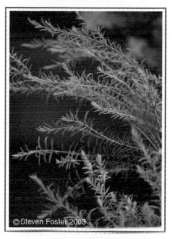

Tea Tree

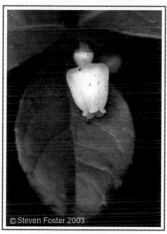

Wintergreen

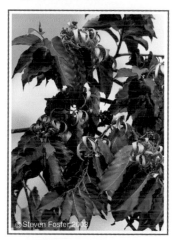

Ylang-Ylang

GERANIUM
Pelargonium graveolens

Known as "women's oil" because of its menstrual and meno-pausal benefits, geranium oil actually has a wide variety of uses. Besides promoting women's health, it's also useful for skin problems like eczema and athlete's foot, and for respira-tory tract health. Its spicy, exotic, floral scent also makes it a fabulous aphrodisiac. Additionally, geranium oil is very gentle and may be used by almost anyone, anywhere, anytime.

THERAPEUTIC USES

Acne, aphrodisiac, athlete's foot, chilblains, circulatory issues, cold sores, cellulite, dandruff, eczema, excess mucous, frostbite, headaches, menopause, mood swings, mosquito repellent, ner-vous tension, PMS symptoms, respiratory issues, sore throat, stress, and tonsillitis.

ESSENTIAL OIL APPLICATIONS

- As an aphrodisiac, add 8 to 10 drops to 1 tablespoon of shower gel, shampoo, or Castile soap and mix into bath water, or use 2 to 3 drops in a diffuser.

- For acne, athlete's foot, chilblains, dandruff, or eczema, place 2 to 3 drops on a cotton ball and dab on affected areas.

- For cellulite, symptoms of menopause, or PMS symptoms, add 20 drops to 1 ounce of carrier oil and massage into body. For cellulite, massage into affected areas. For symptoms of menopause or PMS symptoms, massage into abdominal area and back, paying extra attention to the lower back region.

- For cold sores, place 1 drop on a cotton swab and dab on affected areas.

- For frostbite, massage affected area with approximately 5 drops of oil.

- For headaches, add 8 to 10 drops to 1 tablespoon of shower gel, shampoo, or Castile soap and mix into bath water.

- For nervous tension or stress, use 2 to 3 drops in a diffuser. May also add 2 to 3 drops to 1 ounce of carrier oil for a relaxing massage. For nervous tension or stress that interferes with a good night's rest, put 4 drops on a tissue or cotton ball and place inside pillow case.

- For respiratory issues or excess mucous, use 5 drops in a diffuser.

- For sore throat or tonsillitis, use 2 to 5 drops in a steam inhalation.

- To balance mood, use 2 to 3 drops in a diffuser, or place on a cotton ball or handkerchief and inhale deeply 2 to 3 times.

- To repel mosquitoes, use 5 drops in a diffuser. May also be mixed with citronella for a stronger repellent.

MIXES WELL WITH: Allspice, basil, bergamot, cinnamon, citronella, clove, frankincense, ginger, grapefruit, hyssop, jasmine, juniper berry, lavender, lemon, lime, myrrh, neroli, nutmeg, orange, palmarosa, patchouli, pennyroyal, peppermint, rose, rosemary, rosewood, clary sage, sandalwood, tangerine, tea tree, thyme, and ylang-ylang.

EXTRACTION METHOD: Steam distillation.

PARTS USED: Leaves, stalks, and flowers.

SAFETY INFORMATION: Geranium oil is perfectly safe for home use in moderation. In very large quantities, it may cause irritation to sensitive skin.

FUN FACT

Geraniums used to be planted outside houses to keep evil spirits away.

(See color photo on page 78.)

GINGER

Zingiber officianale

Although its natural appearance might seem a little strange, ginger is one of the most highly valued spices in the world. Not only does it give food a unique spicy, peppery flavor, but it is also renowned for its healing properties. For centuries, different cultures worldwide have embraced it and sung its praises. Traditional Chinese medicine employed fresh ginger to treat a variety of health issues, from respiratory challenges to toothaches. The Greeks used it to counteract the effects of poison. King Henry VIII of England recommended the use of ginger to combat the Great Plague of the sixteenth century. These days, aromatherapists use its warming and soothing qualities to combat digestive and joint complaints and mood swings, as well as to help increase libido.

THERAPEUTIC USES

Arthritis, back pain, chills, circulatory issues, colds, decongestant, digestive issues, flu, libido, lymphatic system, mood swings, muscle pain, rheumatism, runny nose, sinusitis, and sore throat.

ESSENTIAL OIL APPLICATIONS

- For arthritis, back pain, muscle pain, or rheumatism, add 2 to 3 drops to 1 ounce of carrier oil and massage into affected areas. May also use 2 to 3 drops in a hot or cold compress.

- For chills or circulatory issues, add 2 to 3 drops to 1 ounce of carrier oil and massage into body.

- For mood swings, use 2 to 3 drops in a diffuser, or place on a cotton ball and inhale 2 to 3 times. This will help reenergize and revitalize mind, body, and soul.

- For runny nose, sore throat, or sinusitis, or as a decongestant, use 2 to 3 drops in a steam inhalation.

- To boost libido, add 2 to 3 drops to 1 ounce of carrier oil and use as massage oil, or diffuse 2 to 3 drops into air.

- To stimulate the lymphatic system, place a couple of drops on a cotton ball and dab on the armpit area.

MIXES WELL WITH: Allspice, cedarwood, cinnamon, clove, eucalyptus, geranium, grapefruit, jasmine, juniper berry, lemon, lime, myrrh, orange, palmarosa, patchouli, rose, rosemary, sandalwood, spearmint, tangerine, tea tree, and ylang-ylang.

EXTRACTION METHOD: Steam distillation.

PARTS USED: Unpeeled, dried, ground root.

SAFETY INFORMATION: Although it is frequently administered to pregnant women to help alleviate morning sickness, it is best to avoid the use of ginger during pregnancy in aromatherapy practices. For people with extremely sensitive skin, dilute oil carefully before using in massage or bath.

FUN FACT

To rev up their husbands' libidos, the women of Senegal have been known to wear belts with ginger woven into them.

GRAPEFRUIT

Citrus paradisi

Grapefruit is a bit of a botanical mystery. It appears to be a hybrid of a sour fruit known as a shaddock and a sweet orange. There are no existing records to show that there was a deliberate hybridization of these two plants, however, so it remains a mystery as to whether it was deliberately bred or is a product of natural hybridization. Although grapefruit was first cultivated in the West Indies back in the eighteenth century, the United States is now the world's largest producer of grapefruit anywhere. Therapeutically, grapefruit has energizing and cleansing properties, plus it has a unique ability to aid in fat dissolution.

THERAPEUTIC USES

Acne, antiseptic, arthritis, cellulite, depression, disinfectant, fatigue, fluid retention, headaches, mental or nervous exhaustion, menstruation, menstrual cramps, muscle stiffness, rheumatism, and stress.

ESSENTIAL OIL APPLICATIONS

- For acne, place 2 to 3 drops on a cotton ball and dab on affected areas. If you have highly sensitive skin, dilute with carrier oil.

- For arthritis, fatigue, rheumatism, or stiffness, add 2 to 3 drops to 1 ounce of carrier oil and massage into affected areas. May also add 4 to 5 drops to 1 tablespoon of shower gel, shampoo, or Castile soap and mix into bath water, or use in a hot compress.

- For depression, headaches, mental or nervous exhaustion, or stress, use 2 to 3 drops in a diffuser, or place 2 to 3 drops on a handkerchief and periodically inhale.

- To get rid of germs, add 5 to 6 drops to 1 quart of water and pour into a spray bottle. Shake well before using.

- To purify air and kill airborne germs, use 2 to 3 drops in a diffuser.

- To relieve menstrual cramps, add 2 to 3 drops to 1 ounce of carrier oil and massage into lower back and abdominal area. May also be used in a hot compress.

- To stimulate delayed menstruation, add 2 to 3 drops to 1 ounce of carrier oil and massage into lower abdominal area.

MIXES WELL WITH: Basil, cinnamon, clove, eucalyptus, frankincense, geranium, ginger, hyssop, jasmine, juniper berry, lavender, lime, myrrh, neroli, orange, palmarosa, patchouli, peppermint, rosemary, rosewood, sage, clary sage, sandalwood, tangerine, thyme, and ylang-ylang.

EXTRACTION METHOD: Cold expression.

PARTS USED: Fresh peel.

SAFETY INFORMATION: Avoid contact with direct sunlight for twelve hours after use. Grapefruit oil has a short shelf life, as it oxidizes quickly. Replace quarterly.

FUN FACT

In many parts of the world, the waste of grapefruit and other citrus fruits is ground up and used as animal feed.

(See color photo on page 78.)

HELICHRYSUM

Helichrysum italicum

Helichrysum italicum is sometimes called the "curry plant" due to the scent of its leaves, although its flavor is more akin to mild rosemary. *Helichrysum* essential oil is not widely known, but it has been gaining recognition thanks to research showing its ability to lower inflammation and its role as an antimicrobial agent. Named after the golden yellow flowers of the plant, the genus name comes from the Greek words "helix," meaning spiral, and "khrusos," meaning gold. As its flowers last a long time and do not wither easily, this plant is also goes by the names "Immortelle" and "Everlasting."

THERAPEUTIC USES

Acne, after-sun tonic, antibacterial, antifungal, blemishes, bruises, colds, cough, skin inflammation, wounds, and wrinkles.

ESSENTIAL OIL APPLICATIONS

- As an after-sun tonic, place 2 to 3 drops on a cotton ball and apply to skin.

- For colds or cough, use 2 to 3 drops in a diffuser, or add 2 to 3 drops to 1 ounce of carrier oil and rub into chest. May also place 2 to 3 drops on a cotton ball or handkerchief and inhale periodically.

- For blemishes, bruises, skin inflammation, wounds, or wrinkles, add 2 to 3 drops to 1 ounce of carrier oil and apply to affected areas.

MIXES WELL WITH: Bergamot, black pepper, chamomile, citrus oils, clary sage, clove, cypress, geranium, juniper berry, lavender, neroli, oregano, palmarosa, rose, rosemary, tea tree, thyme, vetiver, and ylang-ylang.

EXTRACTION METHOD: Steam distillation.

PARTS USED: Flowers.

SAFETY INFORMATION: *Helichrysum* oil is nontoxic but should not be used on children under twelve years old.

FUN FACTS

Helichrysum was used by the ancient Greek soldiers for its ability to heal wounds.

In addition to its therapeutic uses, *Helichrysum* oil is also thought to promote spiritual growth and compassion.

HYSSOP
Hyssopus officinalis

Hyssop, also known as the holy herb, is mentioned numerous times in the Bible. Used by powerful biblical leaders such as David, Moses, Solomon, and Jesus, hyssop cleansed and purified mankind, both internally and externally. It was also used to wash and polish sacred places. Others embraced hyssop as well. Greeks used hyssop for respiratory problems. Persians used hyssop in a type of body lotion to give skin a fine color. Indians used it to reduce body tissue fluids, alleviate bruises, and soothe cuts and wounds. Europeans in the seventeenth century used hyssop as an air freshener. Once used extensively across the globe, its use in the Western world diminished as modern-day medicine took its place. These days, thanks to a wider acceptance of holistic therapies, hyssop is again a therapeutic leader.

THERAPEUTIC USES

Antiseptic, anxiety, appetite loss, asthma, bloating, bronchitis, bruises, circulatory issues, colds, concentration, cough, creativity, cuts, digestive issues, eczema, emotional balance, excess phlegm, fatigue, flu, low blood pressure, meditation, menstrual problems, nervous tension, skin inflammation, sore throat, stress, tonsillitis, whooping cough, and wounds.

ESSENTIAL OIL APPLICATIONS

- As an antiseptic, place 2 to 3 drops on a cotton ball and apply to wounds.

- For anxiety, fatigue, nervous tension, or stress, or to aid in clarity, concentration, creativity, or meditation, use 2 to 3 drops in a diffuser.

- For appetite loss, bloating, or digestive issues, add 2 to 3 drops to 1 ounce of carrier oil and massage into abdominal area.

- For bronchitis, cough, excess phlegm, or other respiratory problems, use 2 to 3 drops in a diffuser, or add 2 to 3 drops to 1 ounce of carrier oil and massage into chest. May also place 2 to 3 drops on a cotton ball or handkerchief and inhale periodically.

- For cuts, skin inflammation, or wounds, dilute with water, place 2 drops on a cotton ball, and dab on affected areas.

- For emotional balance, use 2 to 3 drops in a diffuser.

- For low blood pressure, use 3 to 5 drops in a diffuser regularly.

- For menstrual problems such as bloating or water retention, add 2 to 3 drops to 1 ounce of carrier oil and massage into lower abdominal area and lower back. May also add 8 to 10 drops to 1 tablespoon of shower gel, shampoo, or Castile soap and mix into bath water.

- For sore throat, tonsillitis, or whooping cough, use 3 to 5 drops in a steam inhalation.

- To boost circulation, add 4 to 6 drops to 2 ounces of carrier oil and massage into entire body.

MIXES WELL WITH: Geranium, grapefruit, lavender, lemon, lime, orange, sage, rosemary, clary sage, and tangerine.

EXTRACTION METHOD: Steam distillation.

PARTS USED: Leaves and flowering tops.

SAFETY INFORMATION: Avoid if pregnant or nursing. Do not use if diagnosed with epilepsy or high blood pressure.

FUN FACT

In the tenth century, Benedictine monks introduced hyssop to Europe as an ingredient for liqueurs.

(See color photo on page 78.)

JASMINE
Jasminum officinale

Exotic and sweet, jasmine is a highly sought after oil. Exorbitantly expensive in its pure form, it's not uncommon to find "cut" or synthetic versions on the market. These variants are beneficial as well as affordable. Jasmine's use goes back centuries. In ancient India, jasmine was (and still is) used for ceremonial purposes. The Chinese used jasmine to cleanse the atmosphere that surrounded the sick. A good hostess also made sure to have jasmine on hand to give to inebriated guests to clear their heads. Modern uses for jasmine include depression, respiration, and fertility.

THERAPEUTIC USES

Confidence, cough, depression, fertility, labor, lack of energy, lactation, libido, menstrual pain, muscle spasms, muscle sprains, nervous tension, optimism, postnatal depression, respiratory issues, skin care, and vitality.

ESSENTIAL OIL APPLICATIONS

- For cough, especially the lingering kind, use 3 to 5 drops in a steam inhalation.

- For depression or nervous tension, use 3 to 5 drops in a diffuser. May also add 8 to 10 drops to 1 tablespoon of shower gel, shampoo, or Castile soap and mix into bath water.

- For menstrual pain, add 8 to 10 drops to 1 tablespoon of shower gel, shampoo, or Castile soap and mix into bath water.

- For muscle spasms or muscle sprains, add 3 to 5 drops to 1 ounce of carrier oil and massage into affected areas.

- For nervous tension or stress, use 2 to 3 drops in a diffuser. May also add 20 drops to 1 ounce of carrier oil and massage into body.

- For postnatal depression, add 3 to 5 drops to 1 ounce of carrier oil and massage into body. May also add 8 to 10 drops to 1 tablespoon of shower gel, shampoo, or Castile soap and mix into bath water, or use 3 to 5 drops in a diffuser.

- For respiratory issues, use 5 drops in a steam inhalation. Especially good for deepening breathing and calming spasms of the bronchi.

- To help strengthen contractions during childbirth and relieve labor pain, use 3 to 5 drops in a diffuser placed in birthing room. Do not start diffusing oil until labor is well advanced.

- To promote libido in both men and women, use 3 to 5 drops in a diffuser, or add 8 to 10 drops to 1 tablespoon of shower gel, shampoo, or Castile soap and mix into bath water.

- To promote male fertility, use regularly in massage (3 to 5 drops added to 1 ounce of carrier oil). May also add 8 to 10 drops to 1 tablespoon of shower gel, shampoo, or Castile soap and mix into bath water, or use 3 to 5 drops in a diffuser.

- To restore confidence, energy, optimism, or vitality, use 3 to 5 drops in a diffuser. May also add 8 to 10 drops to 1 tablespoon of shower gel, shampoo, or Castile soap and mix into bath water.

- To use as a skin tonic for all skin types, mix a few drops with an application of unscented face lotion. May also mix with lavender, tangerine, and carrier oil for a blend that can encourage cell growth and increase elasticity.

- When lactating, jasmine will help promote the flow of breast milk. Add 8 to 10 drops to 1 tablespoon of shower gel, shampoo, or Castile soap and mix into bath water. May also add 3 to 5 drops to 1 ounce of carrier oil and use as massage oil, or use 3 to 5 drops in a diffuser.

MIXES WELL WITH: Bergamot, clove, frankincense, geranium, ginger, grapefruit, lemon, lime, neroli, orange, palmarosa, rose, rosewood, clary sage, sandalwood, tangerine, and ylang-ylang.

EXTRACTION METHOD: Solvent extraction of the flowers can produce both a concrete and an absolute. Jasmine essential oil is produced from the absolute via steam distillation.

PARTS USED: Flowers.

SAFETY INFORMATION: Avoid during most of pregnancy; do not use until labor is well advanced.

(See color photo on page 78.)

JUNIPER BERRY
Juniperus communis

Juniper berry was one of the first aromatics used by ancient civilizations and has a colorful history. Ancient Greeks burned juniper branches to combat epidemics. The English burned it as well, hoping its magical powers would repel evil spirits, witches, and demons. Ancient Egyptians anointed corpses with juniper oil and used the berries in cosmetics and perfumes. Europeans regarded juniper oil as a miracle cure for typhoid, cholera, dysentery, and tapeworms. Many cultures today also value juniper's many benefits. Tibetans still revere juniper and use it as purification incense, while Native Americans burn it in their cleansing ceremonies. Holistic medicine also embraces juniper and considers it highly versatile and therapeutic.

THERAPEUTIC USES

Acne, anxiety, appetite regulator, arthritis, cellulite, colds, disinfectant, eczema, flu, gout, hair loss, headaches, immune system health, infections, insomnia, menstrual regulation, mental exhaustion, nervous tension, oily skin, rheumatism, stress, and wounds.

ESSENTIAL OIL APPLICATIONS

- As a home disinfectant, add 5 drops to 1 quart of water and pour into a spray bottle. Shake well before using.

- For acne, eczema, oily skin, or wounds, place enough oil on a cotton ball to make it wet but not soaked. Wipe directly on skin condition, using gentle movements.

- For anxiety, insomnia, mental exhaustion, nervous tension, or stress, add 8 to 10 drops to 1 tablespoon of shower gel, shampoo, or Castile soap and mix into bath water. May also use 2 to 3 drops in a diffuser.

- For arthritis or rheumatism, add 2 to 3 drops to 1 ounce of carrier oil and massage into affected areas.

- For cellulite, add 2 to 3 drops to 1 ounce of carrier oil and massage into affected areas regularly. May also add 8 to 10 drops to 1 tablespoon of shower gel, shampoo, or Castile soap and mix into bath water.

- For colds or flu, use 3 to 5 drops in a steam inhalation. May also add 8 to 10 drops to 1 tablespoon of shower gel, shampoo, or Castile soap and mix into bath water, or use 3 to 5 drops in a diffuser.

- For hair loss, mix 3 to 5 drops in unscented conditioner. Leave on hair for 3 to 5 minutes and then rinse as normal. Use regularly.

- For headaches, use 2 to 3 drops in a diffuser, or add 8 to 10 drops to 1 tablespoon of shower gel, shampoo, or Castile soap and mix into bath water. May also add 2 to 3 drops to 1 ounce of carrier oil and massage gently into temples. Increase benefit by adding lavender.

- For immune system health, add 8 to 10 drops to 1 tablespoon of shower gel, shampoo, or Castile soap and mix into bath water, or use 2 to 3 drops in a diffuser.

- To regulate appetite, use 2 to 3 drops in a diffuser, or use in a steam inhalation.

- To regulate menstruation and fight menstrual cramps, add 2 to 3 drops to 1 ounce of carrier oil and massage into lower abdominal area.

MIXES WELL WITH: Bergamot, cedarwood, eucalyptus, geranium, ginger, grapefruit, lavender, lime, myrrh, orange, palmarosa, peppermint, pine needle, rosemary, clary sage, sandalwood, tangerine, and tea tree.

EXTRACTION METHOD: Steam distillation.

PARTS USED: Dried, crushed, or slightly dried ripe fruit.

SAFETY INFORMATION: Avoid if pregnant or nursing. Do not use if diagnosed with kidney problems.

(See color photo on page 78.)

LAVENDER
Lavandula angustifolia

Lavender is the most loved aromatic used in aromatherapy today. Besides being versatile in its usage, it has a lightly floral and soothing scent that most people find appealing. In therapeutic terms, lavender is the most useful oil, and one that every aromatherapy kit should include. It's also one of the few essential oils that can be applied neat—using only the oil itself. (Essential oils are highly concentrated plant oils. Read and follow instructions for use carefully.) Lavender has a long history of use in many different cultures but is probably most associated with the English for its use in many of their perfumes.

THERAPEUTIC USES

Acne, alopecia, anxiety, asthma, bee or wasp stings, bronchial issues, depression, dermatitis, eczema, flu, hay fever, headaches, insect repellent, insomnia, menstrual regulation, migraines, minor cuts or burns, mood swings, nervous tension, nightmares, psoriasis, rashes, stress, and sunburn.

ESSENTIAL OIL APPLICATIONS

- For skin problems, including acne, dermatitis, eczema, psoriasis, rashes, and sunburn, place 2 to 3 drops on a cotton ball and dab on affected areas.

- For alopecia, mix 2 to 3 drops in a quarter-sized application of unscented, leave-on conditioner and massage into scalp.

- For headaches or migraines, massage a couple of drops into temples. May also use in a hot or cold compress.

- To relieve insomnia, use 2 to 3 drops in a diffuser, or put 2 to 3 drops on a cotton ball or handkerchief and place inside pillowcase. May also add 8 to 10 drops to 1 tablespoon of shower gel, shampoo, or Castile soap and mix into bath water before bedtime.

- For anxiety, depression, mood swings, nervous tension, or stress, use 2 to 3 drops in a diffuser. May also add 8 to 10 drops to 1 tablespoon of shower gel, shampoo, or Castile soap and mix into bath water. To guard against nightmares, add 8 to 10 drops to 1 tablespoon of shower gel, shampoo, or Castile soap and mix into bath water before bedtime.

- For menstrual regulation, add 4 to 5 drops to 1 ounce of carrier oil and massage into abdominal area and lower back.

- For bee or wasp stings, place 2 to 3 drops on a cotton ball and dab on affected areas.

- For flu, use 2 to 3 drops in a diffuser or steam inhalation.

- To repel moths, put several drops on cotton balls and place in infested areas.

- For asthma, bronchial issues, or hay fever, use 2 to 3 drops in a diffuser or steam inhalation. May also add 4 to 5 drops to 1 ounce of carrier oil and massage into chest area, or add 8 to 10 drops to 1 tablespoon of shower gel, shampoo, or Castile soap and mix into bath water.

MIXES WELL WITH: Almost all oils, but particularly with allspice, anise seed, basil, bergamot, chamomile, citronella, clove, eucalyptus, frankincense, geranium, grapefruit, hyssop, jasmine, juniper berry, lemon, lime, patchouli, peppermint, pine needle, rose, rosemary, clary sage, spearmint, tangerine, tea tree, and thyme.

EXTRACTION METHOD: Steam distillation.

PARTS USED: Fresh flowering tops.

SAFETY INFORMATION: Avoid if pregnant or nursing. May irritate skin. May make those with low blood pressure drowsy.

(See color photo on page 78.)

SPIKE LAVENDER
Lavandula latifolia

Spike lavender has many of the same therapeutic uses as traditional lavender oil (*Lavandula angustifolia*), but unlike the latter, it also contains a significant concentration of camphor that makes it beneficial in the treatment of cough and congestion. This difference is due to the low altitude at which spike lavender grows, which is in contrast to the high elevations at which traditional lavender may be found. Spike lavender oil is also widely employed throughout the fragrance industry, specifically in the manufacture of soap. As you might imagine, the scent of spike lavender is a combination of traditional lavender's sweet floral fragrance and the sharp, medicinal aroma of camphor.

THERAPEUTIC USES

Acne, alopecia, anxiety, asthma, bee or wasp stings, bronchial issues, congestion, cough, depression, dermatitis, eczema, flu, hay fever, headaches, insect repellent, insomnia, menstrual regulation, migraines, minor cuts or burns, mood swings, nervous tension, nightmares, psoriasis, rashes, stress, and sunburn.

ESSENTIAL OIL APPLICATIONS

▦ For alopecia, mix 2 to 3 drops in a quarter-sized application of unscented, leave-on conditioner and massage into scalp.

▦ For anxiety, depression, mood swings, nervous tension, or stress, use 2 to 3 drops in a diffuser. May also add 8 to 10 drops to 1 tablespoon of shower gel, shampoo, or Castile soap and mix into bath water. To guard against nightmares, add 8 to 10 drops to 1 tablespoon of shower gel, shampoo, or Castile soap and mix into bath water before bedtime.

▦ For asthma, bronchial issues, or hay fever, use 2 to 3 drops in a diffuser or steam inhalation. May also add 4 to 5 drops to 1 ounce of carrier oil and massage into chest area, or add 8 to 10 drops to 1 tablespoon of shower gel, shampoo, or Castile soap and mix into bath water.

- For bee or wasp stings, place 2 to 3 drops on a cotton ball and dab on affected areas.

- For cough and congestion, use 2 to 3 drops in a diffuser or steam inhalation. May also add 4 to 5 drops to 1 ounce of carrier oil and massage into chest area, or add 8 to 10 drops to 1 tablespoon of shower gel, shampoo, or Castile soap and mix into bath water.

- For flu, use 2 to 3 drops in a diffuser or steam inhalation.

- For headaches or migraines, massage a couple of drops into temples. May also use in a hot or cold compress.

- For insomnia, use 2 to 3 drops in a diffuser, or put 2 to 3 drops on a cotton ball or handkerchief and place inside pillowcase. May also add 8 to 10 drops to 1 tablespoon of shower gel, shampoo, or Castile soap and mix into bath water before bedtime.

- For menstrual regulation, add 4 to 5 drops to 1 ounce of carrier oil and massage into abdominal area and lower back.

- For skin problems, including acne, dermatitis, eczema, psoriasis, rashes, and sunburn, place 2 to 3 drops on a cotton ball and dab on affected areas.

- To repel moths, put several drops on cotton balls and place in infested areas.

MIXES WELL WITH: Almost all oils, but particularly with allspice, anise, basil, bergamot, chamomile, citronella, clove, eucalyptus, frankincense, geranium, grapefruit, hyssop, jasmine, juniper berry, lemon, lime, patchouli, peppermint, pine needle, rose, rosemary, clary sage, spearmint, tangerine, tea tree, and thyme.

EXTRACTION METHOD: Steam distillation.

PARTS USED: Fresh flowering tops.

SAFETY INFORMATION: Avoid if pregnant or nursing. May irritate skin. May make those with low blood pressure drowsy.

LEMON

Citrus limon

Lemons have long been valued for more than just lemonade. We know that ancient Egyptians prized this oil for its purported ability to act as an antidote to poisoning from meat or fish. And, like lime, it was a staple on seventeenth-century Royal Navy ships to help prevent scurvy. Today, we know lemon can help contain and treat infectious diseases, especially colds and fevers. Its scent also helps neutralize unpleasant odors. Some hospitals use lemon oil to calm frightened or depressed patients. It also boosts the immune system by stimulating production of white and red blood cells. Lemon oil is a must for every aromatherapy kit.

THERAPEUTIC USES

Air freshener, anemia, circulatory issues, colds, constipation, corns, cough, dandruff, depression, digestive issues, fatigue, fever, flu, high blood pressure, household cleanser, immune system health, insect repellent, joint pain, lack of energy, listlessness, mouth ulcers, nail strengthener, nosebleeds, oily hair, oily skin, PMS symptoms, scars, stress, throat infections, voice loss, and warts.

ESSENTIAL OIL APPLICATIONS

- For anemia or high blood pressure, use 2 to 3 drops in a diffuser regularly. May also use in a steam inhalation.

- For circulatory issues, add 2 to 3 drops to 1 ounce of carrier oil and massage into body. May also add 8 to 10 drops to 1 tablespoon of shower gel, shampoo, or Castile soap and mix into bath water, or use a few drops in a steam inhalation.

- For colds, cough, flu, or voice loss, use 2 to 3 drops in a steam inhalation. Also add to carrier oil and massage into chest and neck. To cool a fever, use 2 to 3 drops in a cold compress. After an illness, use 2 to 3 drops in a diffuser or steam inhalation as a tonic for the immune system. Continue use for 2 to 3 days.

- For corns or warts, use neat—that is using only the oil itself—on a cotton swab and apply directly to affected areas. Be careful not to apply to surrounding area.

- For digestive issues, use 2 to 3 drops regularly in a steam inhalation or diffuser.

- For fatigue, PMS symptoms, or stress, use 2 to 3 drops in a diffuser. May also add 8 to 10 drops to 1 tablespoon of shower gel, shampoo, or Castile soap and mix into bath water.

- For joint pain, add 2 to 3 drops to 1 ounce of carrier oil and massage into affected areas. May also add 8 to 10 drops to 1 tablespoon of shower gel, shampoo, or Castile soap and mix into bath water.

- For mouth ulcers or throat infections, use in mouthwash. Swish, gargle, and then rinse with water. Use regularly until condition has abated.

- For nosebleeds, place a few drops on a cotton ball and inhale.

- For oily hair, mix 2 to 3 drops with unscented shampoo. For oily skin, add 2 to 3 drops to 1 ounce of water. Mix well and place on cotton ball. Apply to skin as a toner.

- For scars, add 2 to 3 drops to 1 ounce of carrier oil and massage into affected areas regularly.

- To freshen air or neutralize bad odors, use 2 to 3 drops in a diffuser. While cleaning, add 2 to 3 drops to rinse water to wipe away greasy residue and for extra freshness.

- To repel insects, use 2 to 3 drops in diffuser, or put a few drops on cotton balls and place in infested areas.

- To strengthen nails, add 2 to 3 drops to 1 ounce of almond oil and massage into cuticles and nails regularly.

MIXES WELL WITH: Chamomile, eucalyptus, frankincense, geranium, juniper berry, lavender, neroli, rose, sandalwood, and ylang-ylang.

EXTRACTION METHOD: Cold expression.

PARTS USED: Outer part of fresh peel.

SAFETY INFORMATION: May irritate skin. Avoid direct sunlight after use, as it may have a mild phototoxic effect.

(See color photo on page 79.)

LEMONGRASS
Cymbopogon citratus

Closely related to palmarosa and citronella, lemongrass is a fragrant tropical grass that is native to tropical Asia. For many years, it has been used in Asian cuisine to flavor soups, curries, seafood, and other dishes, but it offers more than just culinary benefits. It is well known for its inclusion in deodorizing sprays and has a refreshing and uplifting aroma. Lemongrass essential oil is also employed frequently as an ingredient in bug repellant. In terms of personal health, it may be added to carrier oil and used to boost circulation, soothe muscle pain, or ease headaches. It is even known to alleviate jet lag!

THERAPEUTIC USES

Acne, air freshener, athlete's foot, excessive perspiration, flatulence, headaches, insect repellent, jet lag, muscle pain, oily skin, scabies, and stress.

ESSENTIAL OIL APPLICATIONS

- For acne or oily skin, add 2 to 3 drops to 1 ounce of carrier oil and gently apply to affected areas several times a day.

- For athlete's foot, muscle pain, or scabies, add 2 to 3 drops to 1 ounce of carrier oil and massage into affected areas several times a day.

- For excessive perspiration, add 2 to 3 drops to 1 ounce of carrier oil and dab on armpits or other affected areas.

- For flatulence, add 2 to 3 drops to 1 ounce of carrier oil and massage into lower abdominal area.

- For headache, add 2 to 3 drops to 1 ounce of carrier oil and massage into temples.

- For jet lag or stress, use 2 to 3 drops in a steam inhalation.

- To freshen air or neutralize bad odors, use 2 to 3 drops in a diffuser.

- To repel insects, use 2 to 3 drops in diffuser, or put a few drops on cotton balls and place in infested areas.

MIXES WELL WITH: Basil, bergamot, black pepper, cedarwood, coriander, cypress, geranium, ginger, grapefruit, lavender, lemon, marjoram, orange, palmarosa, patchouli, rosemary, clary sage, tea tree, thyme, vetiver, and ylang-ylang.

EXTRACTION METHOD: Steam distillation.

PARTS USED: Grass.

SAFETY INFORMATION: Avoid if pregnant or nursing. Avoid if you have kidney or liver disease. Do not use on children under two years old. May cause skin irritation.

FUN FACTS

In the Caribbean, lemongrass is known as "sweet rush" and is used to treat the common cold and fever.

Lemongrass is a perennial plant with a lifespan of approximately four years.

LIME
Citrus aurantifolia

Fruity and refreshing, limes have been a kitchen staple for centuries. It is believed that limes were first introduced to the Americas by sixteenth-century Portuguese navigators. The lime soon became a favorite fruit, both for its taste and therapeutic value. Traditionally, lime has been used as a remedy for indigestion, heartburn, and nausea. It also has cooling effects on fevers and can help ease a cough. Lime oil is also useful as part of a beauty regimen, as its astringent properties help clear oily skin and acne. Plus, because lime oil promotes good circulation, it is often used to help relieve varicose veins. Last but not least, lime oil has a wonderfully uplifting scent, with the power to reenergize the spirit.

THERAPEUTIC USES

Acne, arthritis, cellulite, colds, congestion, cough, cuts, deodorant, depression, disinfectant, fever, general cleaning, immune system health, listlessness, mental exhaustion, nail growth, rheumatism, sinusitis, sore throat, varicose veins, and wounds.

ESSENTIAL OIL APPLICATIONS

- After an illness, use 2 to 3 drops in a diffuser or steam inhalation as a tonic for the immune system. Continue use for 2 to 3 days.

- As a deodorant, add 2 to 3 drops to 1 ounce of water. Dab on with a cotton ball. For extra protection, mix 2 drops in unscented shower gel and shower as normal.

- As a disinfectant, add 5 to 6 drops to 1 quart of water and pour into a spray bottle. Shake well before using.

- For acne, add 2 to 3 drops to 1 ounce of water. Mix well and then place on a cotton ball. Gently apply to affected areas. May also be used as a toner for oily skin.

- For arthritis or rheumatism, add 2 to 3 drops to 1 ounce of carrier oil and massage into affected areas.

- For bleeding cuts or wounds, use 2 to 3 drops in a cold compress.

- For cellulite, add 2 to 3 drops to 1 ounce of carrier oil and massage into affected areas regularly.

- For colds, congestion, cough, sinusitis, or sore throat, use 2 to 3 drops in a steam inhalation. May also be added to carrier oil and massaged into chest and neck.

- For depression, listlessness, or mental exhaustion, use 2 to 3 drops in a diffuser. May also add 8 to 10 drops to 1 tablespoon of shower gel, shampoo, or Castile soap and mix into bath water.

- For varicose veins, add 2 to 3 drops to 1 ounce of carrier oil and massage into affected areas.

- To cool fever, use 2 to 3 drops in a cold compress.

- To promote nail growth, add 2 to 3 drops to 1 ounce of almond oil and massage into cuticles.

- While cleaning refrigerator, freezer, or oven, add 2 to 3 drops to rinse water for extra freshness in wiping away greasy residue.

MIXES WELL WITH: Basil, bergamot, citronella, eucalyptus, geranium, ginger, grapefruit, hyssop, jasmine, juniper berry, lavender, neroli, nutmeg, rosemary, rosewood, sage, sandalwood, tangerine, and ylang-ylang.

EXTRACTION METHOD: Cold expression or steam distillation.

PARTS USED: Peel of unripe fruit (cold expression), whole ripe crushed fruit (steam distillation).

SAFETY INFORMATION: May cause photosensitivity in strong sunlight. Use in moderation.

(See color photo on page 79.)

MARJORAM
Origanum majorana

Its fresh, warm, and slightly woody aroma reflects the meaning of marjoram's botanical name, "joy of the mountains." This popular herb has been used therapeutically for centuries. Ancient Greeks used it to soothe muscle aches, relieve excess fluid in tissues, and as an antidote to poison. Greek women also applied oil with added marjoram on their heads as a relaxant. In sixteenth-century Europe, this herb was scattered on floors of rooms everywhere to mask unpleasant smells. Today, while marjoram may be best known for lending a unique flavor to food, it's also a favorite of aromatherapists. With therapeutic properties that may be used against a number of ailments, including anxiety and high blood pressure, marjoram is a valuable and pleasing aromatic to have on hand.

THERAPEUTIC USES

Anxiety, arthritis, asthma, bronchitis, bruises, chilblains, colds, constipation, cough, digestive issues, flatulence, grief, headaches, high blood pressure, hyperactivity, indigestion, insomnia, lumbago, menstrual cramps, migraines, muscle aches, muscle sprains, muscle stiffness, nervous tension, PMS symptoms, rheumatism, seasickness, and stress.

ESSENTIAL OIL APPLICATIONS

- For anxiety, grief, hyperactivity, insomnia, nervous tension, or stress, use 2 to 3 drops in a diffuser, or add 8 to 10 drops to 1 tablespoon of shower gel, shampoo, or Castile soap and mix into bath water before bedtime.

- For arthritis, lumbago, muscle aches, muscle sprains, muscle stiffness, or rheumatism, add 2 to 3 drops to 1 ounce of carrier oil and massage into affected areas. May also be used in a hot or cold compress.

- For asthma, bronchitis, colds, or cough, add 2 to 3 drops to 1 ounce of carrier oil and massage into chest and throat. May also use 2 to 3 drops in a steam inhalation.

- For bruises or chilblains, add 2 to 3 drops to 1 ounce of carrier oil and dab on affected areas. May also be used neat—that is using only the oil itself—but just on affected areas. (Essential oils are highly concentrated plant oils, therefore always read and follow instructions for use carefully.)

- For digestive issues such as constipation, indigestion, or flatulence, add 2 to 3 drops to 1 ounce of carrier oil and massage into back.

- For headaches or migraines, add 2 to 3 drops to 1 ounce of carrier oil and massage into temples and neck. May also be used in a hot or cold compress.

- For high blood pressure, add 2 to 3 drops to 1 ounce of carrier oil and use in a full-body massage. May also add 8 to 10 drops to 1 tablespoon of shower gel, shampoo, or Castile soap and mix into bath water.

- For menstrual cramps or other PMS symptoms, add 2 to 3 drops to 1 ounce of carrier oil and massage into lower abdominal area and lower back. May also add 8 to 10 drops to 1 tablespoon of shower gel, shampoo, or Castile soap and mix into bath water.

- For seasickness, place 2 to 3 drops on a handkerchief and inhale periodically.

MIXES WELL WITH: Bergamot, cedarwood, cinnamon, eucalyptus, lavender, lemon, orange, pine needle, tangerine, rosemary, rosewood, clary sage, tea tree, thyme, and ylang-ylang.

EXTRACTION METHOD: Steam distillation.

PARTS USED: Fresh and dried leaves and flowering tops.

SAFETY INFORMATION: Avoid if pregnant or nursing. Not suitable for small children. If diagnosed with depression, do not use, as it has a strong, sedative effect. Excessive use may cause drowsiness.

(See color photo on page 79.)

MYRRH

Commiphora myrrha

Best known for its presentation as a gift to the baby Jesus, myrrh appears several more times in the Bible. Myrhh has been used therapeutically for over three thousand years and continues to be a powerhouse in the world of holistic medicine. Ancient Egyptians used myrrh to treat herpes and hay fever. Myrrh was also important to Greek soldiers, who took myrrh into the battlefield with them for its antiseptic and anti-inflammatory properties, which made it helpful for cleaning and healing wounds. Even today, healers all over the world are still using it. Tibetans use myrrh to help alleviate stress and nervous disorders, while the Chinese use it for sores and hemorrhoids. Warm, rich, and spicy in scent, myrrh is a welcome addition to every aromatherapy kit.

THERAPEUTIC USES

Anger, appetite, asthma, athlete's foot, bedsores, boils, bronchitis, chapped skin, colds, cough, digestive issues, eczema, fungal infections, gingivitis, hemorrhoids, mature complexions, mouth ulcers, rheumatism, skin ulcers, sore throat, sores, spongy gums, stress, wounds, and wrinkles.

ESSENTIAL OIL APPLICATIONS

- For anger and stress, use 2 to 3 drops in a diffuser.

- For appetite or digestive issues, use 2 to 3 drops in a diffuser or steam inhalation. May also add 2 to 3 drops to 1 ounce of carrier oil and massage into abdominal area.

- For asthma, colds, cough, or sore throat, add 2 to 3 drops to 1 ounce of carrier oil and massage into chest for asthma, coughs, or cold, and into throat if it is sore. May also use 2 to 3 drops in a diffuser or steam inhalation.

- For athlete's foot, bedsores, boils, fungal infections, skin ulcers, sores, or wounds, use 2 to 3 drops in a cold compress and apply to affected areas. May also be added to a cotton ball and dabbed on directly. Use lightly.

- For chapped skin or hemorrhoids, add 2 to 3 drops to 2 tablespoons of liquid lanolin and massage into affected areas.

- For mouth disorders such as gingivitis, mouth ulcers, or spongy gums, add 2 to 3 drops to a glass of water, swish in mouth, and then spit out.

- To rejuvenate mature complexions and smooth wrinkles, wash face, add 2 to 3 drops to 1 ounce of almond carrier oil and then rub gently on face.

MIXES WELL WITH: Allspice, basil, bergamot, clove, frankincense, geranium, ginger, grapefruit, juniper berry, lavender, lemon, nutmeg, palmarosa, patchouli, peppermint, pine needle, rosemary, sandalwood, spearmint, tangerine, tea tree, thyme, and ylang-ylang.

EXTRACTION METHOD: Steam distillation.

PARTS USED: Oleoresin gum.

SAFETY INFORMATION: Avoid if pregnant or nursing. Do not use in high concentrations.

FUN FACT

According to Greek mythology, Aphrodite transformed Myrrha, the daughter of the king of Cypress, into a shrub (*Commiphora myrrha*).

(See color photo on page 79.)

NEROLI

Citrus aurantium

Neroli oil is heady, sweet, and floral, and is made from the aromatic blossoms of the orange tree. It's rare to find 100-percent neroli oil, as it's impossible for companies to be able to offer it at a low cost. It takes approximately one thousand pounds of orange blossoms to make one pound of neroli oil. Therefore, it is not unusual to find it "cut" with another oil. This is perfectly acceptable and does not reduce neroli's benefits at all. Used for centuries to combat Plague, fever, and nervousness, neroli is one of the most user-friendly oils there is. It helps regenerate skin cells, improves skin elasticity, and even helps with acne, scarring, and stretch marks. Internally, neroli acts as a natural tranquilizer and can relieve chronic anxiety, depression, and stress. Besides being beloved by aromatherapists all over the globe, neroli is also often used in bridal bouquets, both as a symbol of purity and for its ability to calm nerves.

THERAPEUTIC USES

Acne, antispasmodic, anxiety, aphrodisiac, circulatory issues, depression, headaches, hysteria, insomnia, lethargy, mature skin, menopause, neuralgia, panic, PMS symptoms, scars, stress, and stretch marks.

ESSENTIAL OIL APPLICATIONS

- As an antispasmodic to improve colon problems, diarrhea, or nervous dyspepsia, use 2 to 3 drops in a diffuser, or add 4 to 5 drops to 1 ounce of carrier oil and massage into abdominal area.

- For circulatory issues, add 3 to 4 drops to 1 ounce of carrier oil and massage into body. May also add 8 to 10 drops to 1 tablespoon of shower gel, shampoo, or Castile soap and mix into bath water regularly.

- For acne, wet a cotton ball and then apply a few drops of oil. Dab on affected areas lightly.

- For anxiety, depression, hysteria, lethargy, panic, or stress, use 3 to 4 drops in a diffuser. May also add 8 to 10 drops to 1 tablespoon of shower gel, shampoo, or Castile soap and mix into bath water.

- For headaches or neuralgia, use 3 to 4 drops in a hot or cold compress (whichever works best for you).

- For mature skin, mix a drop or two with an application of an unscented face cream and apply as normal.

- For PMS symptoms, use 3 to 4 drops in a diffuser, or add 8 to 10 drops to 1 tablespoon of shower gel, shampoo, or Castile soap and mix into bath water.

- For scars or stretch marks, mix 3 to 4 drops with liquid lanolin and massage into affected areas.

- For the irritability and tearfulness that can accompany menopause, use 3 to 4 drops in a diffuser, or add 8 to 10 drops to bath water regularly. May also add 3 to 4 drops to 1 ounce of carrier oil and massage into body.

MIXES WELL WITH: Bergamot, frankincense, geranium, grapefruit, jasmine, lavender, lemon, lime, orange, rose, rosemary, sandalwood, tangerine, and ylang-ylang.

EXTRACTION METHOD: Steam distillation or enfleurage.

PARTS USED: Orange blossom petals.

SAFETY INFORMATION: Because of its calming and almost tranquilizing affect, do not use when a clear head is needed or before driving a vehicle or operating other heavy machinery.

(See color photo on page 79.)

NUTMEG
Myristica fragrans

Nutmeg is valued by great cooks everywhere for its versatility in the kitchen. Its nutty, spicy, and slightly sweet taste makes it a valuable ingredient in everything from meat dishes to desserts. So prized was nutmeg that in the Middle Ages the Dutch plotted extreme measures to keep the price high, while the English and French hatched their own counterplots to obtain fertile seeds so they could cultivate it themselves. Besides its culinary uses, nutmeg is also a sought-after aromatic. Romans used it as incense and Egyptians for embalming. Indians found nutmeg to be perfect for intestinal disorders, and Italians found it useful in combating Plague. In the Middle Ages, nutmeg was grated and used with lard as an ointment for hemorrhoids. Today, nutmeg is used in aromatherapy in a variety of ways, from improving circulatory problems to boosting libido.

THERAPEUTIC USES

Appetite, arthritis, bad breath, circulatory issues, digestive issues, fainting spells, gout, hemorrhoids, impotence, libido, muscle pain, nervous tension, and rheumatism.

ESSENTIAL OIL APPLICATIONS

- For arthritis, gout, muscle pain, or rheumatism, add 2 to 3 drops to 1 ounce of carrier oil and massage into affected areas. May also be used in a diffuser.

- For bad breath, use a few drops in water as a mouthwash.

- For circulatory issues, add 2 to 3 drops to 1 ounce of carrier oil and massage into body.

- For digestive issues, add 8 to 10 drops to 1 tablespoon of shower gel, shampoo, or Castile soap and mix into bath water. May also use 2 to 3 drops in a diffuser.

- For hemorrhoids, mix 2 to 3 drops of oil with 2 tablespoons of liquid lanolin. Apply to affected areas. May also add to carrier oil.

- For impotence or to boost libido, add 6 to 8 drops to 1 tablespoon of shower gel, shampoo, or Castile soap and mix into bath water.

- For nervous tension, use 2 to 3 drops in a diffuser, or add 8 to 10 drops to 1 tablespoon of shower gel, shampoo, or Castile soap and mix into bath water.

- To revive someone after a fainting spell, put 2 to 3 drops on a cotton ball or handkerchief and place under nose of the person who fainted.

- To stimulate appetite, use 2 to 3 drops in a diffuser.

MIXES WELL WITH: Bergamot, clove, geranium, lime, myrrh, orange, rosemary, clary sage, tangerine, and tea tree.

EXTRACTION METHOD: Steam or water distillation.

PARTS USED: Dried worm-eaten nutmeg seed (worms eat all the starch and fat content).

SAFETY INFORMATION: Avoid if pregnant or nursing. Very large doses can cause nausea or stupor.

FUN FACT

Yankee peddlers used to sell unsuspecting housewives fake nutmeg whittled from wood, bilking them out of money and leaving town before being found out.

(See color photo on page 79.)

ORANGE
Citrus sinensis

Orange oil is one of the best aromatics for beginners. Besides lending a quality ambiance to any environment, orange oil is basically foolproof to use. It mixes well with many essential oils, softening and warming up the blend. It also has a variety of therapeutic uses, from relaxing mind and spirit to boosting circulation. It's a user-friendly oil and inexpensive to keep on hand. Historically, oranges have been associated with generosity and gratitude, and symbolized innocence and fertility. Native to China and India, oranges are now grown in abundance in the Americas, Israel, and the Mediterranean.

THERAPEUTIC USES

Acne, anxiety, blemishes, boredom, bronchitis, cellulite, chills, chronic fatigue syndrome, colds, constipation, cough, creativity, depression, disinfectant, eczema, fear, fever, flu, fluid retention, gingivitis, joint pain, lethargy, mental exhaustion, mouth ulcers, muscle pain, nervous tension, oily skin, PMS symptoms, psoriasis, seasonal affective disorder, skin care, and stress.

ESSENTIAL OIL APPLICATIONS

- For acne, blemishes, or oily skin, wet a cotton ball and add 2 drops of oil. Dab lightly on affected areas.

- For boredom or lethargy, use 2 to 3 drops in a diffuser.

- For cellulite, add 2 to 3 drops to 1 ounce of carrier oil and massage into affected areas regularly.

- For chronic fatigue syndrome, depression, fear, mental exhaustion, nervous tension, or stress, use 2 to 3 drops in a diffuser or steam inhalation. May also add 8 to 10 drops to 1 tablespoon of shower gel, shampoo, or Castile soap and mix into bath water.

- For colds, cough, or flu, use 2 to 3 drops in a steam inhalation. May also add 2 to 3 drops to 1 ounce of carrier oil and massage into chest.

114

- For constipation, add 2 to 3 drops to 1 ounce of carrier oil and massage into lower back area.

- For fluid retention, add 2 to 3 drops to 1 ounce of carrier oil and massage into lower abdominal area and lower back. May also be massaged into other affected areas.

- For gingivitis or mouth ulcers, place 2 to 3 drops in a glass, add water, and mix. Swish around mouth and then spit out. Repeat as necessary.

- For joint or muscle pain, add 2 to 3 drops to 1 ounce of carrier oil and massage into affected areas. May also be used in a hot compress.

- For PMS symptoms or seasonal affective disorder, use 2 to 3 drops in a diffuser. May also add 8 to 10 drops to 1 tablespoon of shower gel, shampoo, or Castile soap and mix into bath water.

- To cool a fever or warm a chill, use in a compress—cold for a fever, hot for a chill. May also add 8 to 10 drops to 1 tablespoon of shower gel, shampoo, or Castile soap and mix into bath water, or add 2 to 3 drops to 1 ounce of carrier oil and use in a massage.

- To inspire creativity, use 2 to 3 drops in a diffuser.

- To reduce inflammation associated with eczema or psoriasis, add 2 to 3 drops to 1 ounce of carrier oil and massage into affected areas.

MIXES WELL WITH: Almost all essential oils, particularly allspice, anise seed, basil, bergamot, cinnamon, citronella, clove, eucalyptus, frankincense, geranium, ginger, grapefruit, hyssop, jasmine, juniper berry, lemon, marjoram, oregano, neroli, nutmeg, palmarosa, patchouli, rosewood, sage, clary sage, sandalwood, and ylang-ylang.

EXTRACTION METHOD: Cold expression.

PARTS USED: Orange peel.

SAFETY INFORMATION: Do not apply before going out into sunlight. Highly sensitive people should perform a patch test.

(See color photo on page 80.)

OREGANO

Origanum vulgare

Probably best known as a workaholic in the kitchen, oregano also has many valuable therapeutic uses. In fact, it may well have first been used for its curative properties before its seasoning properties were discovered. Ancient Egyptians prized oregano for its ability to disinfect wounds and speed up the healing process. It's also believed that they used it in mummification. Throughout the centuries, oregano has been used to soothe coughs, calm digestive disorders, relax tension, and relieve insomnia. As far as kitchen use, it was the Roman gourmet Apicius who loudly proclaimed oregano to be an important part of his culinary creations, leading it to play an important part in Mediterranean cuisine. When GIs returned from overseas after World War II, they yearned for this Mediterranean staple to be added to their meals. Their insistence on enjoying this herb is what helped make it popular in the United States. Today, oregano not only reigns in the kitchen but also rules in the world of aromatherapy.

THERAPEUTIC USES

Allergies, antiseptic, antiviral, appetite, arthritis, asthma, back pain, bronchitis, carpal tunnel syndrome, cellulite, chronic fatigue syndrome, colds, congestion, flu, fungal infections, headaches, immune system health, indigestion, insomnia, lymphatic circulation, menstruation, menstrual cramps, migraines, muscle pain, muscle sprains, nervous tension, rheumatism, and swelling.

ESSENTIAL OIL APPLICATIONS

- For allergies, asthma, bronchitis, or congestion, add 2 to 3 drops to 1 ounce of carrier oil and massage into chest and throat. May also use 2 to 3 drops in a steam inhalation.

- For arthritis, back pain, carpal tunnel syndrome, muscle pain, or rheumatism, add 2 to 3 drops to 1 ounce of carrier oil and massage into affected areas.

- For cellulite, add 2 to 3 drops to 1 ounce of carrier oil and massage into affected areas regularly.

- For chronic fatigue syndrome, insomnia, or nervous tension, use 2 to 3 drops in a diffuser, or add 8 to 10 drops to 1 tablespoon of shower gel, shampoo, or Castile soap and mix into bath water before bedtime.

- For fungal infections, add 2 to 3 drops to 1 ounce of carrier oil and massage into affected areas. Repeat as needed.

- For headaches or migraines, add 2 to 3 drops to 1 ounce of carrier oil and massage into temples and neck. May also be used in a hot or cold compress.

- For indigestion, add 2 to 3 drops to 1 ounce of carrier oil and massage into chest and abdominal area.

- For muscle sprains or swelling, use 2 to 3 drops in a cold compress.

- To boost immune system after sickness, use 2 to 3 drops in a diffuser.

- To boost lymphatic circulation, add 2 to 3 drops to 1 ounce of carrier oil and massage into body.

- To encourage menstruation or alleviate PMS symptoms, add 2 to 3 drops to 1 ounce of carrier oil and massage into lower abdomen and lower back. May also add 8 to 10 drops to 1 tablespoon of shower gel, shampoo, or Castile soap and mix into bath water.

MIXES WELL WITH: Basil, bergamot, cedarwood, citronella, eucalyptus, lavender, lemon, orange, rosemary, tea tree, thyme, and wintergreen.

EXTRACTION METHOD: Steam distillation.

PARTS USED: Dried herb and leaves.

SAFETY INFORMATION: Avoid if pregnant or nursing. May irritate skin.

(See color photo on page 80.)

PALMAROSA
Cymbopogon martinii

Native to India, palmarosa oil has a rose-like scent, which makes it a popular ingredient in soaps, perfumes, and cosmetics. Palmarosa oil also has a variety of therapeutic uses and is especially beneficial in skin care because of its moisturizing properties. It stimulates cell regeneration and regulates sebum production, giving it age-defying properties. Additionally, palmarosa oil is great for the digestive system and was added to Indian curry dishes and West African meat dishes to kill bacteria and aid digestion. Aromatherapists love palmarosa for its skin conditioning properties and calming floral scent.

THERAPEUTIC USES

Acne, colds, cuts, eczema, fatigue, fever, flu, fungal infections (like athlete's foot), intestinal infections, nervous tension, physical exhaustion, scars, stress, and wounds.

ESSENTIAL OIL APPLICATIONS

▨ For acne, eczema, or fungal infections, add 2 to 3 drops to 1 ounce of carrier oil and use a cotton ball to dab on affected areas. May also be used neat—that is using only the oil itself. (Essential oils are highly concentrated plant oils. Read and follow instructions for use carefully.)

▨ For colds or flu, use 2 to 3 drops in a diffuser.

▨ For cuts or wounds, place 2 to 3 drops on a wet cotton ball and dab gently on affected areas. This method will encourage tissue regeneration and help alleviate scarring.

▨ For fatigue, nervousness, physical exhaustion, or stress, use 2 to 3 drops in a diffuser. May also add 8 to 10 drops to 1 tablespoon of shower gel, shampoo, or Castile soap and mix into bath water, or add 2 to 3 drops to 1 ounce of carrier oil and massage into body.

- For intestinal infections, use 3 to 5 drops in a steam inhalation.

- To cool a fever, use 2 to 3 drops in a cold compress. May also add 8 to 10 drops to 1 tablespoon of shower gel, shampoo, or Castile soap and mix into bath water.

- To stimulate sebum production in dry or mature skin, add 2 to 3 drops to 1 ounce of carrier oil and dab gently on skin. May also be used neat—that is using only the oil itself. (Essential oils are highly concentrated plant oils. Read and follow instructions for use carefully.)

MIXES WELL WITH: Bergamot, cedarwood, clary sage, clove, geranium, ginger, grapefruit, jasmine, juniper berry, lavender, lemon, myrrh, orange, patchouli, rose, rosemary, sandalwood, tangerine, thyme, and ylang-ylang.

EXTRACTION METHOD: Steam or water distillation.

PARTS USED: Fresh or dried grass.

SAFETY INFORMATION: No known contraindications, but it's always best to use a patch test before using on skin.

FUN FACTS

Palmarosa oil is used to flavor tobacco.

Palmarosa oil is also known as "poor man's rose oil" due to the similarity of its scent to that of true rose oils, which are more expensive.

PATCHOULI
Pogostemon cablin

Chances are the word "patchouli" brings to mind hippies, free love, and an era of liberation. Nevertheless, patchouli was used in the East long before the 1970s to scent clothes and linens. In the nineteenth century, the British learned to identify patchouli, as it was used to scent imported fabrics from India. While the musky, earthy scent of patchouli is most associated with fabrics, it has therapeutic properties as well. It's an insect repellent, anti-inflammatory, and antifungal. It provides harmony to the body and spirit, and can even fight off body odor by performing as both a deodorant and antiperspirant. It also has the ability to diminish appetite, making it a friend to dieters all over the globe. Finally, it has the rare distinction of actually improving with age—the older the oil, the fuller the scent. Patchouli: It's not just for hippies anymore.

THERAPEUTIC USES

Acne, antiperspirant, anxiety, athlete's foot or other fungal infections, constipation, dandruff, deodorant, dermatitis, eczema, frigidity, insect bites, insect repellent, impotence, libido, loose skin, oily hair, oily skin, stress, fluid retention, and wounds.

ESSENTIAL OIL APPLICATIONS

- As an antiperspirant or deodorant, place 2 to 3 drops on a cotton ball and dab on armpits.

- For acne, dermatitis, or eczema, add 2 to 3 drops to 1 ounce of carrier oil and dab on affected areas. May also be used neat—that is using only the oil itself. (Essential oils are highly concentrated plant oils. Read and follow instructions for use carefully.)

- For anxiety, add 8 to 10 drops to 1 tablespoon of shower gel, shampoo, or Castile soap and mix into bath water. May also use 2 to 3 drops in a diffuser.

- For athlete's foot or other fungal infections, place 2 to 3 drops on a cotton ball and dab on affected areas.

- For constipation, add 8 to 10 drops to 1 tablespoon of shower gel, shampoo, or Castile soap, and mix into bath water for a nice, long soak.

- For dandruff, mix 2 to 3 drops in unscented conditioner and apply to scalp. Leave on for 3 to 5 minutes and then rinse.

- For fluid retention, add 8 to 10 drops to 1 tablespoon of shower gel, shampoo, or Castile soap and mix into bath water. May also add 2 to 3 drops to 1 ounce of carrier oil and massage into body.

- For insect bites, place 2 to 3 drops on a cotton ball and dab on affected areas.

- For oily skin, place 2 to 3 drops on a wet cotton ball and dab on skin. For oily hair, add 2 to 3 drops to a nickel-sized amount of unscented shampoo. Shampoo as normal and then rinse.

- For stress, use 2 to 3 drops in a diffuser.

- To clean wounds, place 2 to 3 drops on a wet cotton ball and dab affected areas gently.

- To complement a diet and exercise regimen, use 2 to 3 drops in a diffuser regularly to reduce appetite. May also add 8 to 10 drops to 1 tablespoon of shower gel, shampoo, or Castile soap and mix into bath water.

- To repel insects, use 2 to 3 drops in a diffuser. May also be put on cotton balls and placed in infested areas.

- To tighten loose skin, especially after weight loss, add 2 to 3 drops to 1 ounce of carrier oil and massage into body regularly. May also add 8 to 10 drops to 1 tablespoon of shower gel, shampoo, or Castile soap and mix into bath water.

MIXES WELL WITH: Allspice, bergamot, cedarwood, cinnamon, frankincense, geranium, ginger, grapefruit, lavender, orange, myrrh, palmarosa, pine needle, rose, rosewood, clary sage, sandalwood, tangerine, and ylang-ylang.

EXTRACTION METHOD: Steam distillation.

PARTS USED: Non-flower leaves.

SAFETY INFORMATION: May inhibit blood clotting and pose a drug interaction hazard. Can have a sedative effect if used in large amounts. Because patchouli can cause appetite loss, do not use if recovering from illness or battling an eating disorder.

(See color photo on page 80.)

PENNYROYAL
Mentha pulegium

Pennyroyal is a member of the mint family and exudes a fresh, minty, herbaceous scent. While its aroma is actually a bit more powerful than those of other mints, its therapeutic value is actually not as strong. Pennyroyal has been used for a variety of ailments and remains current in the British Herbal Pharmacopoeia, which recommends it for flatulence, intestinal colic, the common cold, delayed menstruation, and gout. Its primary use in today's world of aromatherapy, however, is in pet care. Pennyroyal was a favorite of Roman author Pliny the Elder in the fight against fleas, and it is still used to combat fleas to this day.

THERAPEUTIC USES

Colds, delayed menstruation, excessive perspiration, flatulence, fleas, gout, insect repellent, and intestinal disorders.

ESSENTIAL OIL APPLICATIONS

- For colds, use 2 to 3 drops in a diffuser.

- For delayed menstruation, add 2 to 3 drops to 1 ounce of carrier oil and massage into lower abdominal area. DO NOT USE if there is any chance of pregnancy.

- For excessive perspiration, add 2 to 3 drops to 1 ounce of carrier oil and dab on underarms.

- For flatulence, gout, or intestinal disorders, use 2 to 3 drops in a diffuser.

- To protect your dog or cat from fleas, place a few drops on its collar and wait for it to dry before placing around its neck. May also add 2 to 3 drops to pet shampoo. Be sure to rinse pet thoroughly after shampooing.

To repel insects, put a few drops on cotton balls and place in infested areas. Do not place cotton balls in areas where a pet could easily find them.

MIXES WELL WITH: Citronella, geranium, rosemary, and sage.

EXTRACTION METHOD: Steam distillation.

PARTS USED: Fresh or slightly dried herb.

SAFETY INFORMATION: Avoid completely if pregnant or nursing. May be toxic if ingested.

FUN FACTS

Back in the days of yore, pennyroyal was also known as "pudding grass" for its use in a stuffing made of pennyroyal, honey, and pepper that was often used in hog's pudding.

The pennyroyal plant's lilac-colored flowers are packed tightly in spherical formations that resemble pin cushions.

PEPPERMINT
Mentha piperita

Peppermint is one of the most useful and beloved essential oils. Refreshing, cooling, uplifting, and restorative, peppermint has a variety of therapeutic uses. Used extensively in both Eastern and Western medicine for everything from indigestion to diarrhea, headaches to tired feet, and bad breath to cramps. Peppermint is also a big favorite in the food industry, where it may be found as a flavoring agent in gum, candy, ice cream, and pastries. Peppermint's talents, however, really shine in aromatherapy. Its fresh, comforting scent soothes and relieves all sorts of ailments, both mental and physical.

THERAPEUTIC USES

Apathy, arthritis, asthma, back pain, bad breath, bronchitis, circulatory issues, colds, cough, fainting spells, fatigue, flatulence, flu, headaches, indigestion, intestinal disorders, mental exhaustion, migraines, mouth or gum infections, muscle pain, nasal congestion, nausea, stomach cramps, sunburn, tired feet, travel sickness, and vertigo.

ESSENTIAL OIL APPLICATIONS

- For apathy, fatigue, or mental exhaustion, use 2 to 3 drops in a diffuser.

- For arthritis, back pain, bowel disorders (inflammation, constipation, etc.), headaches, mental exhaustion, muscle pain, stomach cramps, or tired feet, add 3 to 4 drops to 1 ounce of carrier oil and massage into body or affected areas.

- For asthma, bronchitis, coughs, or sinus congestion, use 2 to 3 drops in a steam inhalation. May also be used in a diffuser.

- For bad breath or mouth or gum infections, use as a mouthwash.

- For colds or flu accompanied by headaches, use 2 to 3 drops in a diffuser.

- For indigestion or flatulence, add 2 to 3 drops to 1 ounce of carrier oil and massage into back. May also be used in a compress.

- For fainting spells or vertigo, use 2 to 3 drops on a handkerchief and inhale periodically. May also be used in a diffuser.

- For fever, use 2 to 3 drops in a cold compress.

- For headaches or migraines, use 2 to 3 drops in a diffuser.

- For nausea, use 2 to 3 drops in a diffuser. May also place a couple of drops on a handkerchief and inhale periodically.

- For sunburn, mix 2 to 3 drops with 2 tablespoons of liquid lanolin. Apply to affected areas. May also be used in a cold compress or carrier oil.

- For travel sickness, use 2 to 3 drops on a handkerchief and inhale periodically.

MIXES WELL WITH: Basil, eucalyptus, geranium, grapefruit, juniper berry, lavender, lemon, myrrh, pine, rosemary, spearmint, tea tree, and wintergreen.

EXTRACTION METHOD: Steam distillation.

PARTS USED: Flowering herb.

SAFETY INFORMATION: Avoid if pregnant or nursing. Do not use on babies or small children. May irritate sensitive skin. Do a patch test first before applying in large amounts. Do not use in baths. Should not be used in conjunction with homeopathic remedies, as it will act as an antidote.

PINE NEEDLE
Pinus sylvestris

The fresh scent of pine awakens memories of crisp winter days and holidays past. Pine's uniquely comforting and invigorating scent has been used therapeutically for centuries. Ancient Greeks, Egyptians, and Arabians used pine in religious ceremonies and to treat conditions such as bronchitis, tuberculosis, and pneumonia. Native Americans made a special brew with pine needles, that was consumed to prevent scurvy. Pine-needle mattresses are used even today in the Swiss Alps as a remedy for rheumatism. Pine oil is also a favorite in bath oils and foams (always with carrier), thanks to its fresh, lively scent and its ability to alleviate symptoms of rheumatism.

THERAPEUTIC USES

Asthma, athlete's foot, bronchitis, cellulite, colds, cough, cuts, cystitis, digestive issues, drowsiness, eczema, fatigue, flu, hangover, nasal congestion, nervous exhaustion, prostate issues, psoriasis, rheumatism, scabies, sciatica, smoker's cough, sore throat, and sores.

ESSENTIAL OIL APPLICATIONS

- For asthma, bronchitis, cough (including smoker's cough), or sore throat, use 2 to 3 drops in a steam inhalation. May also use 2 to 3 drops in a diffuser, or add 8 to 10 drops to 1 tablespoon of shower gel, shampoo, or Castile soap and mix into bath water.

- For athlete's foot, cuts, eczema, psoriasis, scabies, sores, or other skin irritations, add 2 to 3 drops to 1 ounce of carrier oil and massage into affected areas.

- For cellulite, add 2 to 3 drops to 1 ounce of carrier oil and massage into affected areas regularly. May also add 8 to 10 drops to 1 tablespoon of shower gel, shampoo, or Castile soap and mix into bath water.

- For colds, flu, sinus congestion, or sore throat, use 2 to 3 drops in a diffuser or steam inhalation. May also add 8 to 10 drops to 1 tablespoon of shower gel, shampoo, or Castile soap and mix into bath water.

- For cystitis or prostate issues, add 8 to 10 drops to 1 tablespoon of shower gel, shampoo, or Castile soap and mix into bath water.

- For digestive problems, use 2 to 3 drops in a steam inhalation. May also add 2 to 3 drops to 1 ounce of carrier oil and massage into chest and lower back.

- For drowsiness or nervous exhaustion, use 2 to 3 drops in a diffuser.

- For hangovers, use 2 to 3 drops in a hot or cold compress. May also use 2 to 3 drops in a diffuser, or add 8 to 10 drops to 1 tablespoon of shower gel, shampoo, or Castile soap and mix into bath water.

MIXES WELL WITH: Cedarwood, citronella, eucalyptus, frankincense, grapefruit, juniper berry, lavender, lemon, marjoram, myrrh, patchouli, peppermint, rosemary, sage, clary sage, sandalwood, tea tree, and thyme.

EXTRACTION METHOD: Steam distillation.

PARTS USED: Needles, twigs, and buds.

SAFETY INFORMATION: Avoid if prone to allergic reactions. Avoid if diagnosed with high blood pressure. Should not be used on the skin of children or the elderly. Be sure to avoid oil from *Pinus pumilio* (dwarf pine).

(See color photo on page 80.)

CABBAGE ROSE
Rosa x centifolia

Fragrant, symbolic, and long-lasting, the rose has no equal in beauty or magnificence. It has a long, layered history as rich as its fragrance. The Romans believed roses could prevent drunkenness, so they would scatter the petals at banquets. St. Dominic believed the Virgin Mary had visited him and given him the first rosary, which was made with rose-scented beads. During the Middle Ages, roses were used as an ingredient in various healing balms used to treat ailments such as lung disease and asthma. Also called "provence rose," *Rosa x centifolia* comes predominantly from Egypt, Morocco, and France, and has a sweet aroma with hints of honey.

THERAPEUTIC USES

Allergies, anger, anxiety, asthma, circulatory issues, constipation, cough, depression, digestive issues, grief, hay fever, headaches, irregular menstruation, jealousy, libido, migraines, nausea, nervous tension, postnatal depression, resentment, scars, skin care, sore throat, stress, and vomiting.

ESSENTIAL OIL APPLICATIONS

- For allergies or asthma, use 3 to 4 drops in a diffuser, or add 8 to 10 drops to 1 tablespoon of shower gel, shampoo, or Castile soap and mix into bath water.

- For anxiety or nervous tension, add 2 to 3 drops to 1 ounce of carrier oil and massage into body, or add 8 to 10 drops to 1 tablespoon of shower gel, shampoo, or Castile soap and mix into bath water.

- For circulatory issues, add 3 to 4 drops to 1 ounce of carrier oil and massage into body. May also add 8 to 10 drops to 1 tablespoon of shower gel, shampoo, or Castile soap and mix into bath water.

- For anger, depression, grief, jealousy, or resentment, use 3 to 4 drops in a diffuser.

- For constipation, add 8 to 10 drops to 1 tablespoon of shower gel, shampoo, or Castile soap and mix into bath water.

- For cough or hay fever, add 8 to 10 drops to 1 tablespoon of shower gel, shampoo, or Castile soap and mix into bath water. May also add 3 to 4 drops to 1 ounce of carrier oil and massage into body.

- For headaches or migraines, use 3 to 4 drops in a hot or cold compress (whichever works best for you). May also use 3 to 4 drops in a diffuser.

- For nausea and vomiting, use 3 to 4 drops in a diffuser, or add 8 to 10 drops to 1 tablespoon of shower gel, shampoo, or Castile soap and mix into bath water.

- For overall skin care and to help soften scar tissue, add 2 to 3 drops to 1 ounce of carrier oil and massage into body. May also be mixed with water and applied to face (and is especially good for mature or sensitive skin).

- For postnatal depression, use 3 to 4 drops in a diffuser regularly. May also add 3 to 4 drops to 1 ounce of carrier oil and massage into body regularly.

- To boost libido, add 8 to 10 drops to 1 tablespoon of shower gel, shampoo, or Castile soap and mix into bath water. May also add 2 to 3 drops to 1 ounce of carrier oil and massage into body.

MIXES WELL WITH: Bergamot, cinnamon, clove, frankincense, geranium, ginger, jasmine, lemon, neroli, palmarosa, patchouli, clary sage, sandalwood, tangerine, and ylang-ylang.

EXTRACTION METHOD: Steam distillation or solvent extraction.

PARTS USED: Fresh flower heads.

SAFETY INFORMATION: Avoid if pregnant or nursing.

DAMASK ROSE
Rosa x damascena

The rose has been used to represent transcendent desire in the Sufi tradition and divine love in the Christian tradition. It has also been employed as a symbol in Rosicrucianism, an esteroic cultural movement of the seventeenth century. Touted as very feminine oil, rose oil is excellent for skin care. It's also very expensive. It takes 180 pounds of roses to make 1 ounce of rose oil. Therefore, it is not unusual to find it "cut" with another oil. The benefits will still be in abundance but the cost will be more affordable. Also called "rose of Castile," *Rosa x damascena* is widely grown in Bulgaria and Turkey and has a rich, deep, slightly spicy scent.

THERAPEUTIC USES

Allergies, anger, anxiety, asthma, circulatory issues, constipation, cough, depression, digestive issues, grief, hay fever, headaches, irregular menstruation, jealousy, libido, migraines, nausea, nervous tension, postnatal depression, resentment, scars, skin care, sore throat, stress, and vomiting.

ESSENTIAL OIL APPLICATIONS

- For allergies or asthma, use 3 to 4 drops in a diffuser, or add 8 to 10 drops to 1 tablespoon of shower gel, shampoo, or Castile soap and mix into bath water regularly.

- For anxiety or nervous tension, add 2 to 3 drops to 1 ounce of carrier oil and massage into body, or add 8 to 10 drops to 1 tablespoon of shower gel, shampoo, or Castile soap and mix into bath water.

- For circulatory issues, add 3 to 4 drops to 1 ounce of carrier oil and massage into body. May also add 8 to 10 drops to 1 tablespoon of shower gel, shampoo, or Castile soap and mix into bath water.

- For anger, depression, grief, jealousy, or resentment, use 3 to 4 drops in a diffuser.

- For constipation, add 8 to 10 drops to 1 tablespoon of shower gel, shampoo, or Castile soap and mix into bath water.

- For cough or hay fever, add 8 to 10 drops to 1 tablespoon of shower gel, shampoo, or Castile soap and mix into bath water. May also add 3 to 4 drops to 1 ounce of carrier oil and massage into body.

- For headaches or migraines, use 3 to 4 drops in a hot or cold compress (whichever works best for you). May also use 3 to 4 drops in a diffuser.

- For nausea and vomiting, use 3 to 4 drops in a diffuser, or add 8 to 10 drops to 1 tablespoon of shower gel, shampoo, or Castile soap and mix into bath water.

- For overall skin care and to help soften scar tissue, add 2 to 3 drops to 1 ounce of carrier oil and massage into body. May also be mixed with water and applied to face (and is especially good for mature or sensitive skin).

- For postnatal depression, use 3 to 4 drops in a diffuser regularly. May also add 3 to 4 drops to 1 ounce of carrier oil and massage into body regularly.

- To boost libido, add 6 to 8 drops to 1 tablespoon of shower gel, shampoo, or Castile soap and mix into bath water. May also add 2 to 3 drops to 1 ounce of carrier oil and massage into body.

MIXES WELL WITH: Bergamot, cinnamon, clove, frankincense, geranium, ginger, jasmine, lemon, neroli, palmarosa, patchouli, clary sage, sandalwood, tangerine, and ylang-ylang.

EXTRACTION METHOD: Steam distillation or solvent extraction.

PARTS USED: Fresh flower heads.

SAFETY INFORMATION: Avoid if pregnant or nursing.

(See color photo on page 80.)

ROSEMARY

Rosemarinus officinalis

Rosemary was valued by the ancients of many cultures as a sacred plant that could impart peace to both the living and the dead. The Greeks burnt rosemary at shrines and, along with the Romans, considered it symbolic of remembrance and loyalty. During the Middle Ages, people wore rosemary garlands to bring them good luck and protect them from evil spirits, magic, and witchcraft. It was also thought to help protect against Plague and other infectious illnesses. Nowadays rosemary is a popular culinary herb and used in many delectable dishes. Its charm isn't relegated to the kitchen, though; it's a powerful aromatic as well. Rosemary's fresh, minty, woody aroma can fight fatigue, uplift spirits, renew enthusiasm, and boost self-confidence. Rosemary also has antiseptic properties, making it a strong ally against colds, flu, and respiratory infections. Rosemary is a necessity for every aromatherapy kit.

THERAPEUTIC USES

Acne, antiseptic, arthritis, asthma, back pain, cellulite, colds, constipation, dandruff, depression, diarrhea, enthusiasm, fatigue, flu, fluid retention, headaches, memory, menstrual pain, migraines, muscle pain, nervous exhaustion, oily hair, oily skin, respiratory issues, rheumatism, self-confidence, sinusitis, and stiff neck.

ESSENTIAL OIL APPLICATIONS

▓ For acne or oily skin, place 2 to 3 drops on a wet cotton ball and dab on affected areas.

▓ For arthritis, back pain, muscle pain, rheumatism, or stiff neck, add 2 to 3 drops to 1 ounce of carrier oil and massage into affected areas.

▓ For asthma or respiratory issues, use 2 to 3 drops in a steam inhalation. May also use 2 to 3 drops in a diffuser, or add 8 to 10 drops to 1 tablespoon of shower gel, shampoo, or Castile soap and mix into bath water.

▓ For cellulite, add 2 to 3 drops to 1 ounce of carrier oil and massage into affected areas regularly. May also add 8 to 10 drops to 1 tablespoon of shower gel, shampoo, or Castile soap and mix into bath water.

- For colds or flu, use 2 to 3 drops in a diffuser. May also add 8 to 10 drops to 1 tablespoon of shower gel, shampoo, or Castile soap and mix into bath water.

- For constipation or diarrhea, add 8 to 10 drops to bath water. May also add 2 to 3 drops to 1 ounce of carrier oil and massage into lower back and abdominal area.

- For dandruff or greasy hair, add 2 to 3 drops of oil to unscented conditioner. Leave on for 3 to 5 minutes and then rinse.

- For depression, fatigue, or nervous exhaustion, use 2 to 3 drops in a diffuser.

- For fluid retention, add 8 to 10 drops to 1 tablespoon of shower gel, shampoo, or Castile soap and mix into bath water regularly. May also add 2 to 3 drops to 1 ounce of carrier oil and massage into affected areas regularly.

- For headaches or migraines, especially those related to gastric upset, use 2 to 3 drops in a hot or cold compress. May also use 2 to 3 drops in a diffuser, or add 8 to 10 drops to 1 tablespoon of shower gel, shampoo, or Castile soap and mix into bath water.

- For menstrual pain, add 8 to 10 drops to bath water. May also add 2 to 3 drops to 1 ounce of carrier oil and massage into lower back and abdominal area.

- For sinusitis, use 2 to 3 drops in a steam inhalation.

- To boost enthusiasm, memory, or self-confidence, use 2 to 3 drops in a diffuser.

MIXES WELL WITH: Basil, bergamot, cedarwood, cinnamon, citronella, clove, eucalyptus, geranium, ginger, grapefruit, hyssop, juniper berry, lavender, lemon, lime, marjoram, myrrh, neroli, nutmeg, oregano, palmarosa, pennyroyal, peppermint, pine needle, rosewood, sage, spearmint, tangerine, tea tree, and thyme.

EXTRACTION METHOD: Steam distillation

PARTS USED: Fresh flowering tops or whole plant.

SAFETY INFORMATION: Avoid if pregnant or nursing. Do not use if diagnosed with epilepsy or high blood pressure. Do not rub or massage directly over or below varicose veins.

ROSEWOOD
Aniba rosaeodora

Rosewood is a beautiful, luxurious, amber-colored wood, often made into elegant furniture. The Japanese also use rosewood to make chopsticks. It has a warm, woody, spicy yet floral scent that has made it a favorite component of many perfumes. Additionally, while rosewood may not be one of the most widely used essential oils, it has many highly valued aromatic properties. For centuries, the people of the Amazonian rainforest have used rosewood to heal wounds and for various types of skin ailments. Rosewood can also boost the immune system and relieve headaches. It also has regenerative properties, making it a great tool to use against aging skin, wrinkles, and scars.

THERAPEUTIC USES

Acne, aging skin, colds, cough, physical exhaustion, fever, headaches, infections, insect repellent, lethargy, libido, meditation, nausea, nervous tension, scars, stress, wounds, and wrinkles.

ESSENTIAL OIL APPLICATIONS

- For acne, add 2 to 3 drops to 1 ounce of carrier oil and dab on affected areas.

- For aging skin, scars, or wrinkles, mix 2 to 3 drops with 2 tablespoons of liquid lanolin or a face cream and apply to affected areas.

- For colds or infections, or to boost the immune system in general, use 2 to 3 drops in a diffuser. May also add 8 to 10 drops to 1 tablespoon of shower gel, shampoo, or Castile soap and mix into bath water.

- For physical exhaustion and lethargy, use 2 to 3 drops in a diffuser. For fever, use 2 to 3 drops in a cold compress.

- For headaches, especially those accompanied by nausea, use 2 to 3 drops in a hot or cold compress. May also use 2 to 3 drops in a diffuser, or add 8 to 10 drops to 1 tablespoon of shower gel, shampoo, or Castile soap and mix into bath water.

- For nervous tension, add 2 to 3 drops to 1 ounce of carrier oil and massage into body. May also add 8 to 10 drops to 1 tablespoon of shower gel, shampoo, or Castile soap and mix into bath water.

- For a ticklish cough, use 2 to 3 drops in a steam inhalation. May also add 8 to 10 drops to 1 tablespoon of shower gel, shampoo, or Castile soap and mix into bath water.

- For wounds, use 2 to 3 drops in a cold compress after cleaning wound.

- To boost libido, add 8 to 10 drops to 1 tablespoon of shower gel, shampoo, or Castile soap and mix into bath water. May also add 2 to 3 drops to 1 ounce of carrier oil and massage into body.

- To repel insects, use 2 to 3 drops in a diffuser.

MIXES WELL WITH: Anise seed, cedarwood, geranium, grapefruit, jasmine, lemon, lime, marjoram, orange, patchouli, rosemary, sage, sandalwood, tangerine, tea tree, and ylang-ylang.

EXTRACTION METHOD: Steam distillation.

PARTS USED: Wood chips.

SAFETY INFORMATION: No special precautions.

FUN FACT

Not only is rosewood a favorite among French cabinetmakers, but it is also used to make handles for kitchen utensils.

SAGE
Salvia officinalis

Throughout the ages, sage was considered to be a sacred herb, especially by the Romans, who believed a little sage could cure just about anything. The Chinese also valued sage and believed it to be a cure for sterility. This savory herb found its way into the kitchen and was used to flavor meats and other dishes. As an aromatic, sage has a variety of therapeutic uses, from promoting respiratory health to strengthening memory. Sage is also a popular fragrance in perfumes and colognes, especially men's products. It can also be found in soap, shampoo, detergent, antiperspirant, mouthwash, and toothpaste.

THERAPEUTIC USES

Appetite, arthritis, bronchitis, constipation, cough, fluid retention, indigestion, low blood pressure, memory, menopause, menstruation, over-exercised muscles, respiratory issues, rheumatism, and trauma.

ESSENTIAL OIL APPLICATIONS

▓ For arthritis, over-exercised muscles, or rheumatism, add 2 to 3 drops to 1 ounce of carrier oil and massage into affected areas.

▓ For bronchitis, cough, or other respiratory issues, use 2 to 3 drops in a steam inhalation. May also use 2 to 3 drops in a diffuser.

▓ For constipation, add 8 to 10 drops to 1 tablespoon of shower gel, shampoo, or Castile soap and mix into bath water.

▓ For flatulence, use 2 to 3 drops in a steam inhalation or diffuser.

▓ For indigestion, use 2 to 3 drops in steam inhalation, or add 8 to 10 drops to 1 tablespoon of shower gel, shampoo, or Castile soap and mix into bath water.

- For fluid retention, add 2 to 3 drops to 1 ounce of carrier oil and massage into affected areas. May also add 8 to 10 drops to 1 tablespoon of shower gel, shampoo, or Castile soap and mix into bath water.

- For low blood pressure, use 2 to 3 drops in diffuser or steam inhalation regularly.

- For symptoms of menopause such as hot flashes or night sweats, or to balance nerves, use 2 to 3 drops in a diffuser nightly.

- For scanty periods or painful menstruation, add 8 to 10 drops to 1 tablespoon of shower gel, shampoo, or Castile soap and mix into bath water.

- To boost memory, use 2 to 3 drops in a diffuser regularly.

- To restore a sense of balance and calmness after trauma, especially trauma that continues to haunt you after a long period of time, use 2 to 3 drops in a diffuser nightly until a sense of balance is restored.

- To restore appetite, use 2 to 3 drops in a diffuser.

MIXES WELL WITH: Bergamot, grapefruit, hyssop, lavender, lemon, lime, orange, pennyroyal, pine needle, rosemary, rosewood, and tangerine.

EXTRACTION METHOD: Steam distillation

PARTS USED: Dried leaves

SAFETY INFORMATION: Avoid if pregnant or nursing. If diagnosed with epilepsy or high blood pressure, small amounts are fine, but it would be safest to avoid it. Sage should also not be used on babies or small children.

CLARY SAGE

Salvia sclarea

Clary sage was highly valued during the Middle Ages for its ability to heal all sorts of eye problems. Called "clarus," meaning clear, it was later transformed into clary. Part of its Latin name, *Salvia,* means to save. Rightly so, as clary sage enjoys a reputation as a sort of "cure all" because it has been used to restore health in a variety of areas. Egyptians loved clary sage for its purported ability to cure infertility. Greeks, Romans, and Chinese loved it because they believed it promoted long life. Sixteenth-century Englanders loved it as a replacement for hops to brew beer. Clary sage is also a favorite of creative types, who swear that its fragrance is inspirational. Why not open a bottle yourself and take a whiff? Maybe clary sage will inspire you to greatness!

THERAPEUTIC USES

Anxiety, back pain, depression, digestive issues, insomnia, libido, menopause, muscle pain, neck strain, nervous tension, PMS symptoms, respiratory issues, skin inflammation, and stress.

ESSENTIAL OIL APPLICATIONS

■ For anxiety, decreased libido, depression, insomnia, symptoms of menopause, nervous tension, or stress, use 2 to 3 drops in a diffuser. May also add 2 to 3 drops to 1 ounce of carrier oil and massage into body.

■ For back pain, neck strain, or skin inflammation, mix 2 to 3 drops with 2 to 3 tablespoons of liquid lanolin and apply to problem areas.

■ For respiratory issues, use 2 to 3 drops in a diffuser.

■ For discomfort associated with menopause or premenstrual syndrome, add 4 to 5 drops to 1 tablespoon of shower gel, shampoo, or Castile soap and mix into bath water for a relaxing soak. You may also use 2 to 3 drops on a handkerchief and inhale during times of discomfort. Do not inhale for long periods of time, however, as prolonged exposure could cause headache.

MIXES WELL WITH: Anise seed, bergamot, cedarwood, citrus oils, clove, frankincense, geranium, grapefruit, hyssop, jasmine, juniper berry, lavender, lime, marjoram, nutmeg, palmarosa, patchouli, pine needle, rose, tangerine, tea tree, and thyme.

EXTRACTION METHOD: Steam distillation.

PARTS USED: Flowering tops.

SAFETY INFORMATION: Avoid if pregnant or nursing. Long periods of inhalation could cause headache. Alcohol consumption while using clary sage could increase the effects of alcohol, so it's wise not to imbibe during use.

FUN FACT

Centuries ago, German winemakers added clary sage to inferior wines to make them more intoxicating.

(See color photo on page 80.)

SANDALWOOD
Santalum album

Sandalwood is one of the oldest substances used in perfume and other toiletries with over four thousand years of usage. It has a sensual, musky scent. Besides its presence in many perfumes, sandalwood is also a big part of numerous different types of religious and cultural ceremonies and traditions. Many Muslims burn sandalwood at the feet of the recently deceased to hasten their souls to heaven. In Japan, sandalwood is burned in Shinto ceremonies and at Buddhist shrines, and ancient Egyptians used it in the embalming process. Unfortunately, its popularity has contributed to the fact that sandalwood trees are now almost extinct. They are farmed on plantations exclusively for the production of their essential oil.

THERAPEUTIC USES

Acne, anxiety, aphrodisiac, bladder infections, boils, chapped or dry skin, chest infections, cystitis, dandruff, depression, diarrhea, dry cough, eczema, heartburn, insect repellent, insomnia, nervous tension, razor rash, and sore throat.

ESSENTIAL OIL APPLICATIONS

- As an aphrodisiac, use 2 to 3 drops in a diffuser. May also add 8 to 10 drops to 1 tablespoon of shower gel, shampoo, or Castile soap and mix into bath water.

- For acne, boils, or eczema, add 2 to 3 drops to 1 ounce of carrier oil and dab on affected areas. May also be used neat—that is using only the oil itself. (Essential oils are highly concentrated plant oils. Read and follow instructions for use carefully.)

- For anxiety, depression, insomnia, or nervous tension, use 2 to 3 drops in a diffuser. May also add 8 to 10 drops to 1 tablespoon of shower gel, shampoo, or Castile soap and mix into bath water.

- For chapped or dry skin, mix 2 to 3 drops with 2 tablespoons of liquid lanolin. Rub on affected areas.

- For bladder infections or cystitis, add 8 to 10 drops to 1 tablespoon of shower gel, shampoo, or Castile soap and mix into bath water. May also add 2 to 3 drops to 1 ounce of carrier oil and massage into lower back or abdominal area.

- For chest infections or dry cough, use 2 to 3 drops in a steam inhalation. May also use 2 to 3 drops in a diffuser, or add 8 to 10 drops to 1 tablespoon of shower gel, shampoo, or Castile soap and mix into bath water.

- For dandruff, mix 2 to 3 drops in unscented conditioner and apply to scalp. Leave on for 3 to 5 minutes and then rinse.

- For diarrhea, add 8 to 10 drops to 1 tablespoon of shower gel, shampoo, or Castile soap and mix into bath water for a nice, long soak. May also add 2 to 3 drops to 1 ounce of carrier oil and massage into lower back and abdominal area.

- For heartburn, use 2 to 3 drops to 1 ounce of carrier oil and rub into chest. May also add 8 to 10 drops to 1 tablespoon of shower gel, shampoo, or Castile soap and mix into bath water, or use 2 to 3 drops in a diffuser.

- For razor rash, place 2 to 3 drops on a wet cotton ball and dab on skin.

- For sore throat, apply neat—that is using only the oil itself—to throat area. (Essential oils are highly concentrated plant oils. Read and follow instructions for use carefully.)

- To repel insects, use 2 to 3 drops in a diffuser.

MIXES WELL WITH: Anise seed, basil, bergamot, cedarwood, clove, frankincense, geranium, ginger, grapefruit, jasmine, juniper berry, lavender, lemon, lime, myrrh, neroli, orange, palmarosa, patchouli, pine needle, rose, rosewood, tangerine, and ylang-ylang.

EXTRACTION METHOD: Water or steam distillation.

PARTS USED: Heartwood and roots.

SAFETY INFORMATION: The scent of sandalwood can linger on clothing even after washing.

(See color photo on page 81.)

SPEARMINT

Mentha spicata

Spearmint is a favorite flavor for gums and mints because of its refreshing taste. This herb has been used for centuries, however, for its therapeutic properties as well. Greeks not only used it to scent their bath water but also as a restorative aid. In medieval times, spearmint was used to heal sore gums and whiten teeth. Today, spearmint remains a valued aromatic. It helps with digestive problems, headaches, respiratory issues, and skin problems. Its clean, minty aroma is invigorating and energizing, making it a wonderful scent to come home to after a demanding, stressful day.

THERAPEUTIC USES

Acne, asthma, bronchitis, colds, dermatitis, fatigue, fever, flatulence, flu, headaches, mental exhaustion, migraines, nausea, nervous exhaustion, sinusitis, sore gums, stress, and vomiting.

ESSENTIAL OIL APPLICATIONS

- For acne, add 2 to 3 drops to 1 ounce of carrier oil and dab on affected areas.

- For asthma, bronchitis, or sinusitis, use 2 to 3 drops in a steam inhalation. May also use 2 to 3 drops in a diffuser.

- For colds, fever, or flu, use 2 to 3 drops in a cold compress for fever, or in a hot compress for colds or flu. May also add 8 to 10 drops to 1 tablespoon of shower gel, shampoo, or Castile soap and mix into bath water. Spearmint is also good in a sickroom to help reenergize the ill. Use 2 to 3 drops in a diffuser to help accomplish this task.

- For fatigue, mental exhaustion, nervous exhaustion, or stress, use 2 to 3 drops in a diffuser.

- For flatulence, use 2 to 3 drops in a steam inhalation or diffuser.

- For headaches or migraines, use 2 to 3 drops in a diffuser or steam inhalation. May also use 2 to 3 drops in 1 ounce of carrier oil and massage into temples, or add 8 to 10 drops to 1 tablespoon of shower gel, shampoo, or Castile soap and mix into bath water.

- For sore gums, use in a homemade mouthwash.

- For vomiting, use 2 to 3 drops in a steam inhalation to help calm the system.

MIXES WELL WITH: Basil, eucalyptus, ginger, lavender, myrrh, peppermint, rosemary, and wintergreen.

EXTRACTION METHOD: Steam distillation.

PARTS USED: Fresh flowering tops or whole plant.

SAFETY INFORMATION: Not compatible with homeopathic treatment.

FUN FACT

In ancient times, spearmint was renowned for curing sexually transmitted diseases. Modern medical technology, however, has not proven that spearmint has this power. In other words, kids, don't try this treatment at home.

(See color photo on page 81.)

TANGERINE

Citrus reticulata

Tangerines are much more than a delicious, exotic treat. This fabulous fruit has been used throughout the ages for skin care, digestive health, and system balancing. The warm, sweet, fresh, and lively scent of tangerine is captivating. The French regard tangerine oil as a safe remedy for children suffering from indigestion or hiccups. Tangerine oil is known to inspire, strengthen, and uplift. This essential oil helps combat PMS, promotes healthy digestion, and may reduce scars and stretch marks. It also supports the lymphatic, circulatory, and immune systems. While some may find it similar to orange oil, tangerine oil has its own uniquely comforting and sparkling aroma and should not be replaced by any other citrus oil.

THERAPEUTIC USES

Acne, anxiety, cellulite, constipation, diarrhea, digestive issues, fear, flatulence, hiccups, hyperactivity, insomnia, intestinal disorders, irritability, muscle pain, oily skin, PMS symptoms, restlessness, sadness, scars, stretch marks, and fluid retention.

ESSENTIAL OIL APPLICATIONS

- For acne, oily skin, scars, or stretch marks, add 2 to 3 drops to 1 ounce of carrier oil and massage into affected areas. May also add 8 to 10 drops to 1 tablespoon of shower gel, shampoo, or Castile soap and mix into bath water.

- For anxiety, fear, hyperactivity, insomnia, irritability, PMS symptoms, restlessness, or sadness, use 2 to 3 drops in a diffuser. May also add 8 to 10 drops to 1 tablespoon of shower gel, shampoo, or Castile soap and mix into bath water.

- For cellulite or fluid retention, add 2 to 3 drops to 1 ounce of carrier oil and massage into affected areas regularly. May also add 8 to 10 drops to 1 tablespoon of shower gel, shampoo, or Castile soap and mix into bath water.

- For constipation, diarrhea, or flatulence, add 8 to 10 drops to 1 tablespoon of shower gel, shampoo, or Castile soap and mix into bath water. May also use 2 to 3 drops in a diffuser.

- For digestive issues, add 2 to 3 drops to 1 ounce of carrier oil and gently massage into stomach in a clockwise motion. Do this regularly.

- For hiccups, use 2 to 3 drops in a steam inhalation.

- For muscle pain, add 2 to 3 drops to 1 ounce of carrier oil and massage into affected areas. May also use in a hot compress.

MIXES WELL WITH: Anise seed, basil, bergamot, cinnamon, clove, frankincense, geranium, ginger, grapefruit, hyssop, juniper berry, lavender, lemon, lime, marjoram, myrrh, neroli, nutmeg, palmarosa, patchouli, rose, rosemary, rosewood, sage, clary sage, sandalwood, tea tree, and ylang-ylang.

EXTRACTION METHOD: Cold expression.

PARTS USED: Outer peel.

SAFETY INFORMATION: May be phototoxic; do not use on skin exposed to direct sunlight.

FUN FACT

In the days when gift giving was simpler, tangerines were a favorite stocking stuffer at Christmas.

(See color photo on page 81.)

TEA TREE
Melaleuca alternifolia

Well known for its antiseptic and germicidal properties, tea tree oil has been used therapeutically by Aboriginal Australians for centuries. Named by Captain Cook's crew, it was introduced to Europe around 1927. During World War II, Australian soldiers carried tea tree oil in their first-aid kits as a treatment for skin injuries. Even though tea tree oil has a long history of use therapeutically, it is a relatively new addition to aromatherapy. Despite being the new kid on the block, tea tree oil has become a staple for many aromatherapists around the world because of its versatility and wide-reaching benefits.

THERAPEUTIC USES

Acne, antiseptic, asthma, athlete's foot, blemishes from chicken pox or shingles, blisters, bronchitis, burns, chilblains, cold sores, colds, cough, cracked or dry skin, dandruff, fever, flu, insect bites, recovery from operation, repeated infections, sinusitis, sunburn, varicose veins, warts, and whooping cough.

ESSENTIAL OIL APPLICATIONS

- For acne, athlete's foot, blemishes from chicken pox or shingles, blisters, burns, chilblains, cold sores, cracked or dry skin, dandruff, insect bites, sunburn, varicose veins, or warts, may apply neat—that is using only the oil itself—to affected area (avoid surrounding area). May also be used with water in a compress or in hair rinse. Be sure to carry out a patch test first before applying neat on skin.

- For asthma, bronchitis, cough, sinusitis, or whooping cough, add 8 to 10 drops to 1 tablespoon of shower gel, shampoo, or Castile soap and mix into bath water. May also add 2 to 3 drops to 1 ounce of carrier oil and massage gently into chest and back.

- For colds or flu, use 2 to 3 drops in a diffuser. May also add 8 to 10 drops to 1 tablespoon of shower gel, shampoo, or Castile soap and mix into bath water.

- For fever, use 3 to 5 drops in a cold compress.

- For repeated infections, use 2 to 3 drops in a diffuser regularly. May also add 2 to 3 drops to 1 ounce of carrier oil and massage into body regularly.

- To help prepare the body before an operation, add 2 to 3 drops to 1 ounce of carrier oil and massage into body. To help relieve postoperative shock, use in the same way, carefully avoiding the operation wound or scar.

MIXES WELL WITH: Basil, bergamot, citronella, clove, eucalyptus, geranium, ginger, juniper berry, lavender, lemon, marjoram, myrrh, nutmeg, oregano, peppermint, pine needle, rosemary, rosewood, clary sage, tangerine, tea tree, thyme, and ylang-ylang.

EXTRACTION METHOD: Steam or water distillation.

PARTS USED: Leaves and twigs.

SAFETY INFORMATION: May be used neat—that is using only the oil itself—but it's best to do a patch test first. Limit usage to problem area and avoid surrounding skin. Do not massage directly on or below a varicose vein.

FUN FACT

During World War II, Australian cutters and producers of tea tree oil were exempt from military service until enough of this precious oil had been accumulated for use in first-aid kits.

(See color photo on page 81.)

THYME
Thymus vulgaris

Warm and spicy, thyme has been a beloved aromatic for centuries. Ancient Greeks burned it as incense inside temples. Both Greeks and Romans used thyme to flavor cheese and liquor. Egyptians used it in the embalming process. Thyme was also a symbol of courage, and in the Middle Ages knights wore scarves embroidered with a sprig of thyme. A soup of beer and thyme was once thought to combat shyness. The Scots used to make a tea of wild thyme and believed that drinking it would boost courage and strength as well as prevent nightmares. Now, thyme is most popular in the kitchen, but aromatherapists everywhere know of its therapeutic value and employ it in their practices.

THERAPEUTIC USES

Acne, arthritis, asthma, bronchitis, bruises, burns, chills, circulatory issues, colds, congestion, cough, cuts, dermatitis, eczema, flu, infectious diseases, insect bites, gout, gum infections, headaches, insomnia, laryngitis, muscle aches, muscle pain, muscle sprains, oily skin, physical exhaustion, rheumatism, sinusitis, sore throat, stress, tonsillitis, and warts.

ESSENTIAL OIL APPLICATIONS

- For acne, bruises, burns, cuts, eczema, insect bites, oily skin, or warts, place 2 to 3 drops on a cotton ball and dab on affected areas.

- For arthritis, gout, muscle aches, muscle pain, muscle sprains, or rheumatism, add 2 to 3 drops to 1 ounce of carrier oil and massage into affected areas.

- For asthma, bronchitis, or cough, add 2 to 3 drops to 1 ounce of carrier oil and rub into chest and throat. May also use 2 to 3 drops in a steam inhalation.

- For chills associated with colds or flu, add 2 to 3 drops to 1 ounce of carrier oil and massage into body.

- For circulatory issues, add 2 to 3 drops to 1 ounce of carrier oil and massage into body.

- For colds, flu, congestion, or sinusitis, use 2 to 3 drops in a steam inhalation.

- For gum infections, sore throat, or tonsillitis, use diluted in a gargle or mouthwash.

- For headaches, add 2 to 3 drops to 1 ounce of carrier oil and massage into temples and neck. May also be used in a hot or cold compress.

- For insomnia, physical exhaustion, or stress-related complaints, use 2 to 3 drops in a diffuser.

MIXES WELL WITH: Bergamot, cinnamon, eucalyptus, geranium, grapefruit, lavender, lemon, marjoram, myrrh, oregano, palmarosa, pine needle, rosemary, clary sage, tea tree, and wintergreen.

EXTRACTION METHOD: Steam or water distillation.

PARTS USED: Flowering tops and fresh or partially dried leaves..

SAFETY INFORMATION: Avoid if diagnosed with high blood pressure. Not to be used in baths. Some highly sensitive people could have a reaction, so do a patch test before using neat—that is using only the oil itself—on skin. (Essential oils are highly concentrated plant oils. Read and follow instructions for use carefully.)

FUN FACT

Fairies were once thought to live in beds of thyme. (And who knows for sure? Maybe they do!)

VANILLA
Vanilla planifolia

The scent of vanilla is one of the most popular and recognizable aromas around. It is comforting and sweet, and makes you feel safe and warm instantly. Vanilla essential oil, however, does not exist. The truth is that the vanilla bean does not allow for any of the processes that produce essential oil from a plant. True essential oils must be extracted by physical means only, using no solvents of any kind. But vanilla beans cannot withstand the heat of steam distillation, while mechanical pressing does not yield any oil. Vanilla oil is typically extracted using a solvent, making it, technically, not an essential oil. If you have ever purchased vanilla oil, it was most likely in the form of oleoresin, absolute, or CO_2 extract. The oleoresin type may not mix with carrier oil as well as proper essential oil would, and may leave visible resin in your mixture, while vanilla absolute is much thicker than true essential oil, blends well with other products, but is expensive. The CO_2 extract form, however, will cost you the most to purchase, but it will likely be the most easily blended in carrier oil or diffused.

THERAPEUTIC USES

Anxiety, depression, eczema, insomnia, itching, libido, PMS symptoms, and skin inflammation.

ESSENTIAL OIL APPLICATIONS

- For anxiety or depression, use 2 to 3 drops in a diffuser. May also add 2 to 3 drops to 1 ounce of carrier oil and massage into body where desired.

- For eczema, itching, or skin inflammation, add 2 to 3 drops to 1 ounce of carrier oil and dab on affected areas.

- For insomnia, use 5 to 6 drops in a diffuser. May also place 2 to 3 drops on a tissue and place the tissue inside your pillow before bedtime. Replace nightly.

- For PMS symptoms, add 8 drops to 1 ounce of carrier oil and massage into body regularly.

- To boost libido, use 2 to 3 drops in 1 ounce of carrier oil and use as massage oil, or diffuse 2 to 3 drops into air.

MIXES WELL WITH: Bergamot, frankincense, jasmine, lemon, mandarin, orange, patchouli, rose, sandalwood, vetiver, and ylang-ylang.

EXTRACTION METHOD: Solvent.

PARTS USED: Bean or pod.

SAFETY INFORMATION: Do not take internally.

FUN FACTS

Spanish conquistador Hernán Cortés is credited with introducing both vanilla and chocolate to Europe in the 1520s.

The vanilla orchid requires pollination to produce the seed pods that contain vanilla beans. The flower remains in bloom for only one day, however, and must be pollinated within twelve hours of blooming. It is a difficult task, which explains why vanilla is one of the most expensive spices.

VETIVER
Chrysopogon zizanioides

In Ayurvedic medicine, vetiver oil has been used to treat health-related imbalances and conditions such as arthritis, muscle aches, and headaches for thousands of years. Vetiver essential oil has also been used to sanctify brides before marriage. Vetiver grass is often employed in the making of rugs and baskets. In India, dried vetiver roots are sometimes woven into curtains. When these curtains are sprayed with water, the hot air passing through them creates a cool, aromatic breeze. These days, vetiver oil is mainly used in massage therapy for its ability to settle emotions and calm the mind.

THERAPEUTIC USES

Anxiety, aphrodisiac, arthritis, headaches, insomnia, muscle aches, scars, and termite repellent.

ESSENTIAL OIL APPLICATIONS

- As an aphrodisiac, use 2 to 3 drops in a diffuser, or add 8 to 10 drops to 1 tablespoon of shower gel, shampoo, or Castile soap and mix into bath water.

- For anxiety, use 2 to 3 drops in a diffuser. May also add 2 to 3 drops to 1 ounce of carrier oil and massage into body where desired.

- For arthritis, muscle aches, add 2 to 3 drops to 1 ounce of carrier oil and massage into affected areas.

- For headaches use 2 to 3 drops in a cold compress.

- For insomnia, use 5 to 6 drops in a diffuser. May also place 2 to 3 drops on a tissue and place the tissue inside your pillow before bedtime.

- For scars, add 2 to 3 drops to 1 ounce of carrier oil and dab on affected areas with a cotton ball or swab.

■ To repel termites, add approximately 5 drops to 1 quart of water and pour into a spray bottle. Shake well. Use on affected areas.

MIXES WELL WITH: Bergamot, black pepper, cedarwood, geranium, ginger, grapefruit, jasmine, lavender, lemon, lemongrass, orange, patchouli, rose, clary sage, sandalwood, and ylang-ylang.

EXTRACTION METHOD: Steam distilled.

PARTS USED: Roots.

SAFETY INFORMATION: Do not take internally.

FUN FACT

After Dutch botanist J. F. Veldkamp saw no significant difference between the genus *Chrysopogon* and the genus *Vetiveria*, he reclassified all the grasses in the *Vetiveria* genus to *Chrysopogon*, which had been in use first. Some oil makers still use the *Vetiveria* nomenclature, so don't be confused if you see contrasting identifiers on the market. It's all the same stuff.

WINTERGREEN
Gaultheria procumbens

Traditionally, wintergreen has been used for centuries for sore muscles, arthritis, and rheumatism. While its aroma is on the minty side, it has a warming quality that makes it perfect for relieving the aches and pains associated with these problems. Native Americans used crushed leaves to alleviate the pain of strained muscles and also as an anti-inflammatory. What many may not realize is that wintergreen is often used in perfumery applications, especially fragrances that possess a forest-type scent. And while wintergreen is a well-known flavoring agent in toothpaste, chewing gum, and candy, it is also used in many soft drinks, including root beer and even Coca-Cola.

THERAPEUTIC USES

Acne, arthritis, back pain, cellulitis, fever, fibromylagia, headaches, lumbago, muscle aches, muscle pain, oily skin, rheumatism, sciatica, and sore throat.

ESSENTIAL OIL APPLICATIONS

- For acne or oily skin, add 2 to 3 drops to 1 ounce of carrier oil and dab on affected areas with a cotton ball or swab.

- For arthritis, cellulitis, fibromylagia, lumbago, muscle aches and pain, rheumatism, or sciatica, add 2 to 3 drops to 1 ounce of carrier oil and massage into affected areas.

- For headaches or fever, use 2 to 3 drops in a cold compress.

- For sore throat, add 2 to 3 drops to 1 ounce of carrier oil and massage into throat.

MIXES WELL WITH: Oregano, peppermint, spearmint, thyme, and ylang-ylang.

EXTRACTION METHOD: Steam or water distillation.

PARTS USED: Leaves.

SAFETY INFORMATION: Avoid if pregnant or nursing. Only for topical use, and only if diluted. Avoid using on children under twelve.

FUN FACT

During the Revolutionary War, wintergreen leaves were used as tea because black tea was so highly taxed.

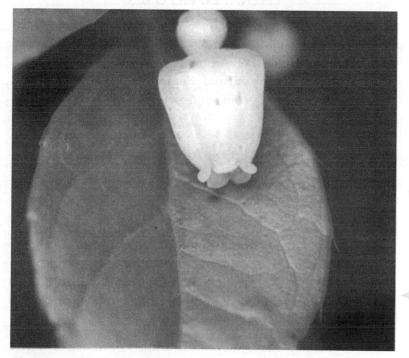

(See color photo on page 81.)

YLANG-YLANG
Cananga odorata

Exotic. Mysterious. Spicy. These three words describe ylang-ylang to a "T." Ylang-ylang's aroma can both uplift and relax. It's been around for centuries and has been most frequently used as an aphrodisiac, yet it has many other stimulating qualities as well. Victorians used it to encourage hair growth. The Chinese used it for circulatory health and to balance the heart. Early twentieth-century researchers discovered that ylang-ylang oil is effective against malaria, typhus, and various intestinal infections. Around the same time, researchers also recognized that ylang-ylang had a calming effect on the heart. Today, ylang-ylang is a treasured essential oil, and is actually more powerful when combined with other oils.

THERAPEUTIC USES

Anxiety, aphrodisiac, circulatory issues, depression, chapped or dry skin, fear, frigidity, hair loss, high blood pressure, impotence, insomnia, intestinal infections or upset, oily skin, panic, physical exhaustion, postnatal depression, rapid breathing, rapid heartbeat, shock, stomach upset or mild food poisoning, and stress.

ESSENTIAL OIL APPLICATIONS

- As an aphrodisiac, use 2 to 3 drops in a diffuser, or add 8 to 10 drops to 1 tablespoon of shower gel, shampoo, or Castile soap and mix into bath water.

- For anxiety, depression, insomnia, panic, physical exhaustion, postnatal depression, rapid breathing or heartbeat, or stress, use 2 to 3 drops in a diffuser. May also add 8 to 10 drops to 1 tablespoon of shower gel, shampoo, or Castile soap and mix into bath water.

- For circulatory issues, add 2 to 3 drops to 1 ounce of carrier oil and massage into body.

- For frigidity or impotence, use 2 to 3 drops in a diffuser, or add 8 to 10 drops to 1 tablespoon of shower gel, shampoo, or Castile soap and mix into bath water.

- For high blood pressure, use 2 to 3 drops in a diffuser or steam inhalation regularly.

- For oily skin, place 2 to 3 drops on a damp cotton ball and apply to affected areas.

- For stomach upset or mild food poisoning, add 2 to 3 drops to 1 ounce of carrier oil and massage gently into stomach.

- To stimulate hair growth, add 2 to 3 drops to 1 ounce of carrier oil and massage into scalp. Leave on for 20 minutes and then shampoo out.

MIXES WELL WITH: Allspice, bergamot, cedarwood, cinnamon, frankincense, geranium, ginger, grapefruit, jasmine, lavender, lemon, lime, marjoram, myrrh, neroli, orange, palmarosa, patchouli, rose, rosewood, sandalwood, tangerine, tea tree, and wintergreen.

EXTRACTION METHOD: Steam or water distillation.

PARTS USED: Fresh, fully developed flowers.

SAFETY INFORMATION: Use in small qualities. Using too frequently or in high doses could cause headaches or nausea in some people. Do not use on inflamed skin or skin affected by dermatitis.

FUN FACT

Indonesians spread ylang-ylang petals
on the beds of newly wedded couples.

(See color photo on page 81.)

Resources

There are numerous companies in the marketplace that create or sell essential oils. Some are more reputable than others. The following are businesses that I am familiar with and trust.

NOW Foods
244 Knollwood Dr
Bloomingdale, IL 60108
Phone: 888-669-3663
Website: www.nowfoods.com

NOW Foods offers both pure (free of synthetic ingredients) and certified organic essential oil products. These oils can be found at health food stores across the country or ordered through any store that carries NOW nutritional supplements. Go to the company's website to find a store near you.

Aroma Vera
Room 303, 3/F
Yan Hing Centre
9-13 Wong Chuk Yeung St
Fo Tan, Hong Kong
Phone: 852-2735-8101
Email: cs@avil.com.hk
Website: www.aromavera.com.hk

With over 100 choices, Aroma Vera essential oils are carried by select retailers and are also sold through catalogs and online. This is a good source for some of the more exotic oils.

AromaLand
1326 Rufina Circle
Santa Fe, NM 87507
Phone: 800-933-5267
Website: www.aromaland.com

AromaLand is a leading source for quality aromatherapy and body care products. It offers one of the largest selections of aromatherapy products in the world in both branded consumer sizes and bulk sizes. AromaLand oils are carried by select retailers and are also sold through catalogs and online.

Aura Cacia
c/o Frontier Co-op
PO Box 299
3021 78th St
Norway, IA 52318
Phone: 844-550-7200
Email: customercare@auracacia.com
Website: www.auracacia.com

Aura Cacia offers essential oils and skin care oils made from simple and pure botanical ingredients. It sources its ingredients carefully and sustainably from the best sources around the world and then tests every shipment of essential oil it receives to verify its purity and quality.

Young Living
Thanksgiving Point Business Park
3125 Executive Parkway
Lehi, UT 84043
Phone: 801-418-8900

Email: custserv@youngliving.com
Website: www.youngliving.com
Using a proprietary production process, Young Living claims to produce the best, most authentic essential oils in the world. The company touts its commitment to creating pure, powerful products for every family and lifestyle.

References

Ali, E., Grant, G., Selim, N., Patel, D., and Ken Vegotsky. *The Tea Tree Oil Bible*. Toronto, ON: Hushion House Publishing Ltd., 1999.

Balch, Phyllis A. *Prescription for Herbal Healing*. New York: Avery, 2002.

Berwick, Ann. *Aromatherapy A Holistic Guide: Balance the Body and Soul with Essential Oils*. St. Paul, MN: Llewellyn, 1994.

Brown, Denise Whichello. *Aromatherapy*. Lincolnwood, IL: NTC Publishing, 1996.

Byers, Dorie. *Natural Beauty Basics: Create Your Own Cosmetics and Body Care Products*. Garden City Park, NY: Square One Publishers, 2007.

Byers, Dorie. *Natural Body Basics: Making Your Own Cosmetics*. Ridgefield, CT: Vital Health Publishing, 1996.

Cooksley, Valerie. *Healing Home Spa*. New York: Prentice Hall Press, 2003.

Dana, Mrs. William Star. *How to Know the Wild Flowers*. Boston: Houghton Mifflin Company, 1989.

Edwards, Victoria H. *The Aromatherapy Companion*. North Adams, MA: Storey Publishing, LLC, 1999.

Fischer-Rizzi, Susanne. *Complete Aromatherapy Handbook: Essential Oils for Radiant Health*. New York, Sterling Publishing Co., 1990.

Gattefossé, René-Maurice. *Gattefossé's Aromatheraphy*. London: C.W. Daniel Co. Ltd., 1937.

Kaminski, Patricia. *Flowers That Heal: How to Use Flower Essences*. Newleaf, 1998.

Lavabre, Marcel. *Aromatherapy Workbook*. Healing Rochester, Vermont. 1990.

Lawless, Julia. *The Illustrated Encyclopedia to Essential Oils: The Complete Guide to the Use of Oils in Aromatherapy and Herbalism*. Shaftesbury, England: Element Books Ltd., 1995.

Lawless, Julia. *Rose Oil*. Great Britain: Thorsons Publishers, 1995.

Metcalfe, Joannah. *Culpepper Guides Herbs and Aromatherapy*. London: Bloomsbury Books, 1989.

Mindell, Earl. *Earl Mindell's Herb Bible*. New York: Fireside Book/Simon & Schuster, 1992.

Nuzzi, Debra. *Pocket Herbal Reference Guide*. Freedom, CA: Crossing Press, 1992.

Richard, David. *Anoint Yourself With Oil for Radiant Health*. Ridgefield, CT: Vital Health Publishing, 1997.

Schiller, Carol & David. *Aromatherapy Oils: A Complete Guide*. New York: Sterling Publishing Co., 1996.

Tisserand, Robert B. *The Art of Aromatherapy*. Rochester, VT: Healing Arts Press. 1978.

Walters, Clare. *Aromatherapy: An Illustrated Guide*. Boston: Element Books Inc., 1998.

Wilson, Roberta. *Aromatherapy: Essential Oils for Vibrant Health and Beauty*. New York: Avery, 2002.

Worwood, Valerie Ann. *The Complete Book of Essential Oils & Aromatherapy*. San Rafael, CA: New World Library, 1991.

About the Author

Mary Shipley has been interested in the field of natural health since the 1970s. After her graduation from Northern Illinois University, Mary went to work at Here's Health natural food store and later became a sales representative at NOW Foods. Through these experiences, she learned extensively about herbs, supplements, and natural medicine. This knowledge led her to help in the development of outstanding standards of quality for the essential oil line of products at NOW Foods. Mary is now retired and living in Iowa, where she continues to be active in growing many of her own herbs to support an aromatic and healthy lifestyle.

Index

Acne, 19, 42, 52, 54, 82, 86, 88, 94, 96, 98
    102, 104, 110, 114, 118, 120, 132
    134, 140, 142, 144, 143, 148, 154
After-Sun, 19, 46, 88
Aging, 19, 74, 134
Aggression, 19, 52. *See also* Anger.
Agitation, 19, 52
Air Freshener, 19, 52, 62, 100, 102
Allergies, 19, 116, 128, 130
Allspice, 34, 76
Alopecia, 19, 96, 98
Anemia, 19, 100
Anger, 20, 52, 108, 128, 130
Anise Seed, 36, 76
Antibacterial, 20, 40, 44, 64, 68, 70,
    72, 88
Antiperspirant, 20, 120. *See also*
    Perspiration, excessive.
Antiseptic, 20, 48, 50, 68, 70, 72, 86,
    90, 116, 132, 146
Antispasmodic, 20, 110. *See also*
    Colitis.
Antiviral, 20, 40, 116
Anxiety, 20, 40, 42, 52, 58, 66, 90, 94,
    96, 98, 106, 110, 114, 120, 128,
    130, 138, 140, 144, 150, 152, 156
Apathy, 20, 124
Aphrodisiac, 20, 82, 110, 140, 152, 156

Appetite, 20, 42, 90, 94, 108, 112, 116,
    120, 136
Arthritis, 20, 38, 40, 44, 50, 52, 54, 60,
    64, 68, 70, 72, 84, 86, 94, 104,
    106, 112, 116, 124, 132, 136, 148,
    152, 154
Aroma families, 9–10
Aromatherapy
    basic, applications, 10–13
    basic, recipes, 10–13
    basis of, 3–6
    grandfather of. *See* Imhotep.
    how to practice, 6–7, 10–14
    how, works, 5–6
    reference guide, 19–33
Aromatic bath, 10–11
Aromatic shower, 11
Asthma, 20, 36, 52, 54, 64, 74, 90, 96,
    98, 106, 108, 116, 124, 126, 128,
    130, 132, 142, 146, 148
Athlete's Foot, 20, 82, 102, 108, 118,
    120, 126, 146
Ayurvedic medicine, 5

Back pain, 21, 84, 116, 124, 132, 138,
    154. *See also* Arthritis;
    Lumbago; Muscle pain; Muscle
    spasms; Muscle sprains.

Bacteria, airborne, 21, 65, 69, 71, 73
Bad breath, 21, 36, 42, 64, 112, 124
Balsam Fir Needle, 38
Basil, 40, 76
Bedsores, 21, 74, 108
Bee stings, 21, 96, 98. *See also* Wasp
    stings.
Bergamot, 42
Black pepper, 44
Bladder infections, 21, 140. *See also*
    Urinary tract health; Urinary
    tract infections.
Bladder issues, 21, 52
Blemishes, 21, 52, 74, 88, 114, 146. *See*
    also Chicken pox; Warts.
Blending oils, 16–17
Bloating, 21, 90. *See also* Fluid
    retention; PMS symptoms.
Blood pressure
    high, 21, 100, 106, 156
    low, 21, 90, 136
Boils, 21, 108, 140
Boredom, 21, 114
Breath
    bad. *See* Bad breath.
    shortness. *See* Shortness of
    breath.
Bronchial issues, 21, 96, 98
Bronchitis, 21, 36, 46, 48, 52, 54, 60,
    64, 66, 74, 90, 106, 108, 114, 116,
    124, 126, 136, 142, 146, 148
Bruises, 21, 46, 88, 90, 106, 148
Burns, minor, 21, 22, 96, 98, 146, 148

Camphor, 46, 76
Care, oil, 17–18
Carpal tunnel syndrome, 22, 116
Carrot Seed, 48
Cassia, 50, 76
Cedarwood, Atlas, 52, 76
Cedarwood, Virginian, 54, 77
Cellulite, 22, 52, 82, 86, 94, 104, 114,
    116, 126, 132, 144

Cellulitis, 22, 154
Chamomile, Maroc, 56
Chamomile, Roman, 58, 77
Chapped skin, 22, 48, 108, 140, 146,
    156. *See also* Dry skin.
Chest infections, 22, 34, 64, 140
Chicken pox, 22, 68, 70, 72, 146
Chilblains, 22, 82, 106, 146. *See also*
    Frostbite.
Childbirth. *See* Labor, childbirth.
Chills, 22, 46, 60, 64, 74, 84, 114, 148
Chronic fatigue syndrome, 22, 114,
    116. *See also* Fatigue.
Cinnamon, 60
Circulatory issues, 22, 44, 60, 66, 74,
    82, 84, 90, 100, 110, 112, 124,
    128, 130, 148, 156
Citronella, 62, 77
Cleanser, household, 22, 100, 104
Clove, 64, 77
Cognitive health, 22, 44, 64
Cold sores, 22, 82, 146
Colds, 22, 34, 36, 40, 42, 46, 48, 50, 52,
    60, 64, 74, 84, 88, 90, 94, 100,
    104, 106, 108, 114, 116, 118, 122,
    124, 126, 132, 134, 142, 146, 148
Colitis, 22, 56
Concentration, 23, 40, 90
Confidence, 23, 92
Congestion, 23, 38, 44, 54, 68, 70, 72,
    74, 84, 98, 104, 116, 124, 126, 148
Constipation, 23, 100, 106, 114, 120,
    124, 128, 130, 132, 136, 144. *See*
    also Digestive issues;
    Indigestion.
Corns, 23, 100
Cough, 23, 34, 46, 52, 54, 66, 68, 70,
    72, 74, 88, 90, 92, 98, 100, 104,
    106, 108, 114, 124, 126, 128, 130,
    134, 136, 140, 146, 148. *See also*
    Colds; Whooping cough.
Cracked skin, 23, 146. *See also*
    Chapped skin.

Creativity, 23, 90, 114

Cramps, stomach. *See* Stomach cramps.

Cuts, minor, 23, 64, 90, 96, 98, 104, 118, 126, 148

Cypress, 66

Cystitis, 23, 42, 52, 54, 74, 126, 140

Dandruff, 23, 52, 54, 82, 100, 120, 132, 140, 146

Decongestant. *See* Congestion.

Deodorant, 23, 104, 120

Depression, 23, 40, 42, 58, 86, 92, 96, 98, 100, 104, 110, 114, 128, 130, 132, 138, 140, 150, 156

postnatal. *See* Postnatal depression.

Dermatitis, 24, 96, 98, 120, 142, 148

Diarrhea, 24, 50, 60, 64, 110, 124, 132, 140, 144

Diffusion, 13

Digestive issues, 24, 34, 36, 42, 44, 48, 60, 62, 84, 90, 100, 106, 108, 112, 124, 126, 128, 130, 138, 144. *See also* Constipation; Heartburn; Indigestion.

Direct application, 12

Disinfectant, 24, 86, 94, 104, 114

Dreams, 24, 36,

Drowsiness, 24, 126

Dry skin, 24, 48, 140, 146, 156. *See also* Chapped skin.

Eczema, 24, 42, 52, 54, 82, 90, 94, 96, 98, 108, 114, 118, 120, 126, 140, 148, 150. *See also* Dermatitis; Psoriasis.

Egypt, 4–5

Emotional balance, 24, 90

Energy, lack of, 24, 92, 100

Enthusiasm, 24, 132

Eucalyptus, Blue Gum, 68, 77

Eucalyptus, Lemon, 70

Eucalyptus, Narrow-Leaved Peppermint, 72

Exhaustion, mental, 24, 64, 86, 94, 104, 114, 124, 142

Exhaustion, nervous, 24, 60, 86, 126, 132, 142

Exhaustion, physical, 24, 118, 134, 148, 156

Fainting spells, 24, 112, 124

Fatigue, 24, 38, 40, 42, 44, 62, 74, 86, 90, 100, 118, 124, 126, 132, 142. *See also* Energy, lack of.

Fear, 25, 114, 144, 156

Fertility, 25, 92

Fever, 25, 42, 100, 104, 114, 118, 134, 142, 146, 154. *See also* Colds; Flu.

Fibromyalgia, 25, 154

Flatulence, 25, 36, 42, 102, 106, 122, 124, 142, 144. *See also* Gas, excess.

Fleas, 25, 62, 122

Flu, 25, 36, 40, 42, 46, 48, 52, 60, 64, 74, 84, 90, 94, 96, 98, 100, 114, 116, 118, 124, 126, 132, 142, 146, 148

Fluid retention, 25, 52, 86, 114, 120, 132, 136, 144. *See also* Bloating.

Food poisoning, mild, 25, 156

Foot or hand bath, 11

Frankincense, 74, 77

Frigidity, 25, 120, 156

Frostbite, 25, 82. *See also* Chilblains.

Fungal infections, 25, 108, 116, 118, 120. *See also* Athlete's foot; Fungus, skin.

Fungus, skin, 25, 52

Gargle, 13

Gas, excess, 25, 44, 58. *See also* Flatulence.

Geranium, 82, 78

Ginger, 84

Gingivitis, 25, 108, 114. *See also* Gum infections; Gums, sore; Gums, spongy; Toothache.
Gout, 25, 94, 112, 122, 148
Grapefruit, 86, 78
Grief, 25, 106, 128, 130
Guide to the uses of essential oils, 19–33
Gum infections, 25, 124, 148. *See also* Gingivitis; Gums, sore; Gums, spongy; Toothache.
Gums, sore, 25, 142. *See also* Gingivitis; Gum infections; Gums, spongy; Toothache.
Gums, spongy, 25, 108. *See also* Gingivitis; Gum infections; Gums, sore; Toothache.

Hair loss, 26, 52, 94, 156. *See also* Alopecia.
Hair, oily, 26, 52, 100, 120, 132
Hangover, 26, 126. *See also* Headaches; Migraines; Nausea.
Hay fever, 26, 96, 98, 128, 130. *See also* Sneezing.
Headaches, 26, 40, 56, 58, 62, 82, 86, 94, 96, 98, 102, 106, 110, 116, 124, 128, 130, 132, 134, 142, 148, 152, 154. *See also* Migraines.
Heartbeat, rapid, 26, 156
Heartburn, 26, 140
Helichrysum, 88
Hemorrhoids, 26, 66, 74, 108, 112
Herpes. *See* Cold sores.
Hiccups, 26, 36, 144
Holistic medicine, 4
Hot or cold compress, 12
Household cleanser. *See* Cleanser, household.
Hyperactivity, 26, 106, 144
Hyssop, 90, 78
Hysteria, 26, 110

Imhotep, 5
Immune system health, 26, 52, 94, 100, 104, 116, 134
Impotence, 26, 112, 120, 156
Indigestion, 26, 106, 116, 124, 136. *See also* Constipation; Digestive issues; Heartburn.
Infections, 26, 42, 94, 134, 146. *See also* Bladder infections; Chest infections; Fungal infections; Gum infections; Intestinal infections, Mouth infections; Throat infections; Urinary tract infections.
Insect bites, 26, 58, 120, 146, 148
Insomnia, 26, 56, 58, 94, 96, 98, 106, 110, 116, 138, 140, 144, 148, 150, 152
Intestinal disorders, 26, 56, 122, 124, 144
Intestinal infections, 26, 60, 118, 156
Irritability, 27, 56, 144

Jasmine, 92, 78
Jealousy, 27, 128, 130
Jet lag, 27, 102
Joint pain, 27, 100, 114. *See also* Arthritis; Lumbago; Rheumatism.
Juniper Berry, 94, 78

Kidney issues, 27, 50, 52, 54

Labor, childbirth, 27, 74, 92. *See also* Lactation; Postnatal depression; Stretch marks.
Lactation, 27, 92
Laryngitis, 27, 74, 148. *See also* Sore throat; Tonsillitis.
Lavender, 96, 78
Lavender, Spike, 98
Lemon, 100, 79

Lemongrass, 102
Lethargy, 27, 110, 114, 134
Libido, 27, 60, 84, 92, 112, 120, 128, 130, 134, 138, 150
Lime, 104, 79
Listlessness, 27, 100, 104
Liver health, 27, 56
Lumbago, 27, 106, 154. *See also* Arthritis; Back pain.
Lymphatic system health, 27, 84, 116

Marjoram, 106, 79
Massage, 13
Meditation, 27, 52, 74, 90, 134
Memory, 27, 132, 136. *See also* Aging.
Menopause, 27, 56, 82, 110, 136, 138
Menstrual health, 27, 40, 74, 86, 90, 94, 96, 98, 116, 122, 128, 130, 136
Menstrual pain, 27, 36, 60, 92, 106, 116, 132
Migraines, 28, 36, 40, 56, 62, 96, 98, 106, 116, 124, 128, 130, 132, 142. *See also* Headaches.
Mood swings, 28, 82, 84, 96, 98
Mouth infections, 28, 42, 124. *See also* Gum infections; Ulcers, mouth.
Mouthwash, 13
Mucous, excess, 28, 82. *See also* Phlegm, excess.
Muscle aches, 28, 36, 38, 44, 48, 106, 148, 152, 154. *See also* Back pain; Muscle pain; Muscle spasms; Muscle sprains; Muscle stiffness.
Muscle pain, 28, 34, 44, 46, 64, 68, 70, 72, 84, 102, 112, 114, 116, 124, 132, 138, 144, 148, 154. *See also* Back pain; Muscle aches; Muscle spasms; Muscle sprains; Muscle stiffness.
Muscle spasms, 28, 40, 64, 92. *See also* Back pain; Muscle aches; Muscle pain; Muscle sprains.
Muscle sprains, 28, 46, 92, 106, 116, 148. *See also* Back pain; Muscle aches; Muscle pain; Muscle spasms; Muscle stiffness.
Muscle stiffness, 28, 86, 106. *See also* Back pain; Muscle aches; Muscle pain.
Myrrh, 108, 79

Nail growth, 28, 104
Nail strength, 28, 100
Nausea, 28, 36, 50, 58, 64, 124, 128, 130, 134, 142
Neck, stiff. *See* Stiff neck.
Neck strain, 28, 138
Neroli, 110, 79
Nervous exhaustion. *See* Exhaustion, nervous.
Nervous tension, 29, 40, 42, 52, 54, 82, 90, 92, 94, 96, 98, 106, 112, 114, 116, 118, 128, 130, 134, 138, 140
Neuralgia, 29, 110
Nightmares, 29, 96, 98
Nosebleeds, 29, 100
Nutmeg, 112, 79

Oily hair. *See* Hair, oily.
Oily skin, 29, 100, 102, 104, 114, 120, 132, 144, 148, 154, 156
Optimism, 29, 92
Orange, 114, 80
Oregano, 116, 80
Organic oil, 17

Palmarosa, 118
Panic, 29, 110, 156
Patchouli, 120, 80
Pennyroyal, 122
Peppermint, 124
Perspiration, excessive, 29, 62, 102,

120, 122. *See also*
Antiperspirant.
Phlegm, excess, 29, 90. *See also*
Mucous, excess.
Pine Needle, 126, 80
PMS symptoms, 29, 58, 82, 100, 106,
110, 114, 138, 144, 150. *See also*
Bloating; Headaches;
Migraines.
Postnatal depression, 29, 92, 128, 130,
156. *See also* Depression.
Prayer, 29, 74
Prostate issues, 29, 126
Psoriasis, 29, 42, 54, 96, 98, 114, 126.
See also Dermatitis; Eczema.
Psychoneuroimmunology, 4

Rapid heartbeat. *See* Heartbeat,
rapid.
Rashes, 30, 96, 98, 140
Reference guide. *See* Guide to the
uses of essential oils.
Repellent, feline, 30, 62
Repellent, insect, 30, 46, 52, 54, 62, 68,
70, 72, 96, 98, 100, 102, 120, 122,
134, 140. *See also* Repellent,
mosquito; Repellent, termite.
Repellent, mosquito, 30, 54, 82
Repellent, rodent, 30, 38
Repellent, termite, 30, 152
Resentment, 30, 128, 130. *See also*
Anger; Anxiety; Nervous
tension; Stress.
Respiratory issues, 30, 38, 40, 52, 54,
60, 64, 66, 68, 70, 72, 82, 84, 90,
92, 104, 132, 136, 138, 142
Restlessness, 30, 144
Rheumatism, 30, 36, 40, 50, 52, 54,
60, 64, 68, 70, 72, 74, 84, 86, 94,
104, 106, 108, 112, 116, 126, 132,
136, 148, 154. *See also* Arthritis;
Joint pain; Lumbago.

Rose, Cabbage, 128
Rose, Damask, 130, 80
Rosemary, 132
Rosewood, 134
Runny nose, 30, 84

Sadness, 30, 144. *See also* Depression;
Postnatal depression.
Sage, 136
Sage, Clary, 138, 80
Sandalwood, 140, 81
Sauna, 11–12
Scabies, 30, 102, 126
Scars, 30, 74, 100, 110, 118, 128, 130,
134, 144, 152
Sciatica, 30, 126, 154
Seasickness, 30, 106
Seasonal affective disorder, 31, 114
Self-confidence, 31, 132
Shingles, 31, 68, 70, 72, 146
Shortness of breath, 21, 74
Sinusitis, 31, 68, 70, 72, 84, 104, 132,
142, 146, 148. *See also* Colds;
Sneezing.
Skin care, 31, 48, 56, 92, 100, 114, 118,
128, 130, 144
Skin inflammation, 31, 58, 88, 90,
138, 150. *See also* Acne;
Dermatitis; Eczema; Fungus,
skin; Psoriasis.
Skin, loose, 31, 120
Skin, oily. *See* Oily skin.
Skin, sensitive, 31, 56
Sleeping aid. *See* Insomnia.
Smoking cessation, 31, 44
Sneezing, 31, 36, 60. *See also* Colds;
Nasal congestion.
Sore throat, 31, 38, 42, 82, 84, 90, 104,
108, 126, 128, 130, 140, 148, 154.
See also Laryngitis; Throat
infections; Tonsillitis.
Sores, 31, 74, 108, 126

Spearmint, 142, 81
Spleen health, 31, 56
Stamina, 31, 44
Steam inhalation, 12
Stiff neck, 31, 132
Stimulant, 32, 44, 48
Stomach cramps, 32, 36, 124. *See also*
    Colitis; Nausea; Seasickness;
    Upset stomach.
Storage, oil, 17–18
Stress, 32, 38, 40, 42, 44, 52, 54, 60, 64,
    66, 82, 86, 90, 92, 94, 96, 98, 100,
    102, 106, 108, 110, 114, 118,
    120, 128, 130, 134, 138, 142, 148,
    156. *See also* Agitation; Anger;
    Anxiety; Resentment.
Stretch marks, 32, 110, 144. *See also*
    Labor, childbirth.
Sunburn, 32, 96, 98, 124, 146
Swelling, 32, 116

Tachycardia. *See* Heartbeat, rapid.
Tangerine, 144, 81
Tea Tree, 146, 81
Throat infections, 32, 68, 70, 72, 100.
    See also Laryngitis; Sore throat;
    Tonsillitis.
Throat, sore. *See* Laryngitis; Sore
    throat; Throat infections;
    Tonsillitis.
Thyme, 148
Tired feet, 32, 124
Tonsillitis, 32, 42, 82, 90, 148. *See also*
    Laryngitis; Sore throat; Throat
    infections.
Toothache, 32, 34, 64. *See also*
    Gingivitis; Gum infections;
    Gums, sore; Gums, spongy.

Trauma, 32, 136
Travel sickness, 32, 124

Ulcers, mouth, 32, 100, 108, 114
Ulcers, skin, 32, 52, 108
Upset stomach, 32, 156. *See also*
    Colitis; Nausea; Seasickness;
    Stomach cramps.
Urinary tract health, 33, 42. *See also*
    Bladder infections; Urinary
    tract infections.
Urinary tract infections, 33, 54, 74. *See
    also* Bladder infections; Urinary
    tract health.

Vanilla, 150
Varicose veins, 33, 66, 104, 146
Vascular disorders, 33, 50
Vertigo, 33, 36, 52, 124
Vetiver, 152
Vitality, 33, 92
Voice loss, 33, 100
Vomiting, 33, 128, 130, 142. *See also*
    Nausea.

Warts, 33, 64, 100, 146, 148. *See also*
    Blemishes.
Wasp stings, 33, 96, 98. *See also* Bee
    stings.
Whooping cough, 33, 36, 90, 146
Wintergreen, 154, 81
Wounds, 33, 42, 48, 58, 74, 88, 90, 94,
    104, 108, 118, 120, 134. *See also*
    Ulcers, skin.
Wrinkles, 33, 48, 88, 108, 134

Ylang-Ylang, 156, 81

Other Square One Titles of Interest

The Healing Power of Rainforest Herbs

A Guide to Understanding and Using Herbal Medicinals

Leslie Taylor, ND

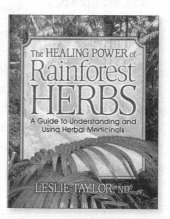

A unique guide to the benefits of rainforest herbs, this book details more than seventy botanicals, presents the history of the herbs' uses by indigenous peoples, and describes current usage by health practitioners. Dosage and preparation methods are provided.

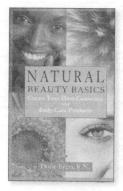

Natural Beauty Basics

Create Your Own Cosmetics and Body Care Products

Dorie Byers, RN

Every day, television and magazine ads tell us that beautiful skin and hair are available only through the use of costly brand-name products. But the fact is that you can attain a radiant appearance by using products made inexpensively at home. That's what *Natural Beauty Basics* is all about. The author guides you to the equipment and ingredients you'll need to make your own products, and then presents easy-to-follow recipes for over 150 all-natural, effective, allergen-free creams, shampoos, soaps, and more.

Apple Cider Vinegar
Nature's Most Versatile and Powerful Remedy

Larry Trivieri, Jr.

Best-selling health author Larry Trivieri, Jr. has written this complete A-to-Z guide that shows how to use apple cider vinegar to prevent and reverse over eighty common health conditions, and to improve and maintain the health and appearance of your hair, skin, teeth, and gums.

$14.95 US • 240 pages • 6 x 9-inch paperback • ISBN 978-0-7570-0446-9

Coconuts for Your Health
Nature's Most Delicious & Effective Remedy

Larry Trivieri, Jr.

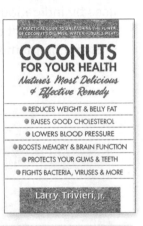

Coconut has been found to raise good cholesterol, reduce belly fat, boost memory, protect teeth and gums, lower blood pressure, and more. This book focuses on specific concerns from heart disease to high blood pressure to memory loss, and explains how coconut works to combat these issues.

$15.95 US • 192 pages • 6 x 9-inch paperback • ISBN 978-0-7570-0451-3

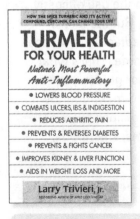

Turmeric for Your Health
Nature's Most Powerful Anti-Inflammatory

Larry Trivieri, Jr.

Turmeric for Your Health is a simple guide to understanding the science behind turmeric's effectiveness. Along with breakthrough research, it presents an A-to-Z listing of ailments for which turmeric can provide successful treatment.

$15.95 US • 192 pages • 6 x 9-inch paperback • ISBN 978-0-7570-0452-0

What You Must Know About Homeopathic Remedies

A Concise Guide to Understanding and Using Homeopathy

Earl Mindell, RPh, MH, PhD

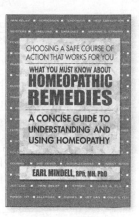

Homeopathy has become a widely accepted way of treating many common disorders. These medicines have no known side effects, are easy to take, and are highly effective. In response to the growing interest in this traditional method of healing, Dr. Earl Mindell has written a simple and concise guide to understanding and using homeopathic remedies. If you are one of the millions of people who are turning to homeopathic products for relief, here is a simple way to find the best formula for your needs.

$9.95 US • 96 pages • 6 x 9-inch paperback • ISBN 978-0-7570-0457-5

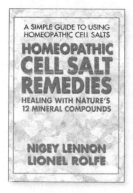

Homeopathic Cell Salt Remedies

Healing with Nature's 12 Mineral Compounds

Nigey Lennon and Lionel Rolfe

In 1870, Dr. W.H. Schuessler, physiological chemist and physicist, developed the use of twelve cell salt remedies in the treatment of illness. Dr. Schuessler discovered that cell salts are essential to maintaining health, and that when the body's stores of these compounds are depleted, we become susceptible to disease. *Homeopathic Cell Salt Remedies* is a comprehensive guide to the theory and use of homeopathic cell salts. Here is a much-needed introduction to the effective use of these important mineral compounds.

$12.95 US • 160 pages • 6 x 9-inch paperback • ISBN 978-0-7570-0250-2

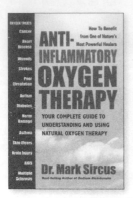

Anti-Inflammatory Oxygen Therapy

Your Complete Guide to Understanding and
Using Natural Oxygen Therapy

Dr. Mark Sircus

This groundbreaking book serves as a guide to oxygen therapy, explaining its use in detoxification and as a treatment for disorders such as arthritis and asthma. Special consideration is given to oxygen therapy as a treatment for cancer.

$15.95 US • 192 pages • 6 x 9-inch paperback • ISBN 978-0-7570-0415-5

Sodium Bicarbonate

Nature's Unique First Aid Remedy

Dr. Mark Sircus

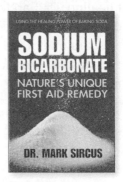

Sodium Bicarbonate begins with an overview of baking soda, chronicling its use as a home remedy. Author Mark Sircus then details how this extraordinary substance can alleviate a number of health disorders and suggests the most effective way to use sodium bicarbonate in the treatment of each condition. Let *Sodium Bicarbonate* help you look at baking soda in a whole new way.

$16.95 US • 208 pages • 6 x 9-inch paperback • ISBN 978-0-7570-0394-3

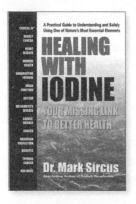

Healing With Iodine

Your Missing Link To Better Health

Dr. Mark Sircus

It is estimated that 90 percent of our population is iodine deficient, and odds are most of us wouldn't think twice about it. This deficiency can directly result in some terrible health problems—from cancer to heart failure to a host of other dreaded diseases. *Healing With Iodine* is a clear guide to understanding and recognizing this missing link to better health.

$16.95 • 176 pages • 6 x 9-inch paperback • ISBN 978-0-7570-0467-4

Juice Alive
SECOND EDITION
The Ultimate Guide to Juicing Remedies

Steven Bailey, ND, and Larry Trivieri, Jr.

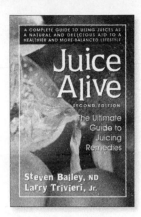

The world of fresh juices offers a powerhouse of antioxidants, vitamins, minerals, and enzymes. The trick is knowing which juices can best serve your needs. In this easy-to-use guide, health experts Dr. Steven Bailey and Larry Trivieri, Jr. share everything you need to know to maximize the benefits of juice. It examines the healthful components of fresh juice, offers practical advice about the types of juices available, and shares tips for buying and storing produce. Rounding out the book are100 delicious juice recipes. Let *Juice Alive* introduce you to the incomparable tastes and benefits of fresh juice.

$14.95 US • 288 pages • 6 x 9-inch paperback • ISBN 978-0-7570-0266-3

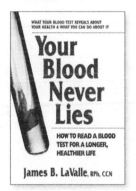

Your Blood Never Lies
How to Read a Blood Test for a Longer, Healthier Life

James B. LaValle, RPh, CCN

Your Blood Never Lies clears the mystery surrounding blood test results. In simple language, Dr. LaValle explains all of the information found on these forms, making it understandable and accessible so that you can look at the results yourself and know the significance of each marker. He even recommends the most effective treatments for dealing with problematic findings and provides the names of test markers that should be requested for a complete physical picture.

$16.95 US • 368 pages • 6 x 9-inch paperback • ISBN 978-0-7570-0350-9

For more information about our books,

visit our website at www.squareonepublishers.com